Sports Cardiology Casebook

Antonio Pelliccia

Editor

Sports Cardiology Casebook

Foreword by Barry J. Maron

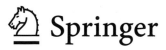 Springer

Editor
Antonio Pelliccia, MD
Institute of Sports Medicine and Science
Italian National Olympic Committee
Rome
Italy
ant.pelliccia@libero.it

ISBN 978-1-84882-041-8   e-ISBN 978-1-84882-042-5
DOI 10.1007/978-1-84882-042-5

British Library Cataloguing in Publication Data
A catalogue record for this book is available from the British Library

Library of Congress Control Number: 2008940853

Printed on acid-free paper

Springer Science+Business Media
springer.com

Foreword

Sudden death in young athletes engaged in competitive sports is a highly visible, emotionally charged and important public health issue, which has increasingly become part of the consciousness of the general public and practicing sports medicine community. Substantial progress has ensued in this new area of cardiovascular medicine since its inception 25 years ago. Indeed, considerable data are now available from both the U.S. and Europe defining the causes, frequency and demographics of these tragic and counterintuitive events which strike to the core of our sensibilities.

There has been a recent focus (and, in fact, controversy) regarding the most effective and appropriate strategies for mass preparticipation screening for the detection of otherwise unsuspected cardiovascular diseases. Finally, given the identification of a cardiovascular abnormality in a trained athlete, several scientific societies, i.e., American College of Cardiology (ACC), European Society of Cardiology (ESC) and Italian Sports Cardiology Society (SIC Sport) have offered detailed guidelines and consensus recommendations which represent criteria with which clinical decisions regarding management and eligibility/disqualification decisions can be effected.

This multi-authored book, the **Sports Cardiology Casebook**, edited by Dr. Antonio Pelliccia, a noted international authority on sports medicine, cardiovascular disease in athletes and chair of the ESC guidelines for eligibility/disqualification, is an important contribution to our understanding of this important and growing area of medicine. Dr. Pelliccia has compiled from international experts several case vignettes illustrating some of the dilemmas implicit in reaching the difficult decisions regarding appropriate recommendations in athletes with underlying cardiovascular disease. These are, invariably situations involving individuals greatly invested in sports, often at elite or professional levels with their livelihood dependent on continued eligibility. In drawing the "line in the sand" between eligibility and disqualification, clinicians can rely in large measure on the aforementioned consensus guidelines. . .but, in the end, a substantial measure of individual clinical acumen is often required. Thus, the Pelliccia book represents a particularly useful addition to the literature in this field which will facilitate clinical practice related to athletes.

Barry J. Maron, MD
Minneapolis Heart Institute Foundation
Minneapolis, Minnesota

Contents

Contributors

Editor:

Antonio Pelliccia, MD Institute of Sports Medicine and Science, Italian National Olympic Committee, Department of Medicine, Largo Piero Gabrielli, 00197 Rome, Italy, ant.pelliccia@libero.it

Co-Editors:

Hein Heidbuchel, MD, PhD Department of Cardiology – Electrophysiology, University Hospital Gasthuisberg, University of Leuven, Leuven, Belgium, hein.heidbuchel@uz.kuleuven.ac.be

Nicole M. Panhuyzen-Goedkoop, MD Department of Sports Cardiology, Sint Maartenskliniek, Sports Medical Centre Papendal, Radboud University, Hospital Nijmegen, Arnhem, The Netherlands, n.panhuyzen@smcp.nl

Authors:

Giuseppe Allocca, MD Cardiology Unit, Conegliano Hospital, Conegliano, Treviso, Italy

Silvana Archetti, PhD Diagnostic Department, A.O. Spedali Civili, Brescia, Italy

Sabrina Arondi, MD Department of Medicine, University of Brescia, Brescia, Italy

Deodato Assanelli, MD Chair of Sport Medicine, Department of Surgical and Medical Sciences, University of Brescia, Montichiari Hospital, Brescia, Italy, assanell@med.unibs.it

Enrico Ballardini, MD Sport Medicine Center, San Pellegrino Hospital, Castiglione delle Stiviere, Mantova, Italy

Sandeep Basavarajaiah, MBBS, MRCP   Essex Cardiothoracic Centre, Department of Cardiology, Basildon, Essex, England

Alessandro Biffi, MD   Institute of Sports Medicine and Science, Italian National Olympic Committee, Department of Medicine, Rome, Italy, alessandro.biffi@coni.it

Massimo Bolognesi, MD   Department of Cardiology, Hospital of Conegliano, Hospital of Santa Maria dei Battuti, Mestre and Conegliano, Italy

Mats Borjesson, MD, PhD   Department of Medicine, Sahlgrenska University Hospital, Östra, Gothenburg, Sweden, mats.brjesson@telia.com

T. Butz, MD   Department of Cardiology, Ruhr University, Bochum, North Rhine-Westphalia, Germany

F. Van Buuren, MHH MD   Heart Center, Department of Cardiology, Bad Oeynhausen, North Rhine-Westphalia, Germany

François Carré, MD, PhD   Department of Physiology, Unité de Biologie.et de Médecine du Sport, Pontchaillou Hospital*,*.Rennes 1 University, INSERM U 642, France, francois.carre@univ-rennes1.fr

Roberto Ciardo, MD   Institute of Sport Medicine and Science, Italian National Olympic Committee, Department of Medicine, Rome, Italy

Leonardo Coro', MD   Department of Cardiology, Hospital of Conegliano, Hospital of Santa Maria dei Battuti, Mestre and Conegliano, Italy

Elvira DeBlasiis, MD   Institute of Sport Medicine and Science, Italian National Olympic Committee, Department of Medicine, Rome, Italy, elvdeb@tin.it

Charles Delagardelle, MD   Hospital Centre of Luxembourg, Department of Cardiology, Luxembourg

Pietro Delise, MD   Department of Cardiology, Ospedale di Conegliano, Hospital of Santa Maria dei Battuti, Mestre and Conegliano, Italy, pietro.delise@libero.it

Mikael Dellborg, MD, PhD   Department of Medicine, Sahlgrenska University Hospital, Östra, Gothenburg, Sweden

Federica Ettori, MD   Cardiology Division, Spedali Civili, Brescia, Italy

Laura Fiaccarini   Institute of Sports Medicine and Science, Italian National Olympic Committee, Department of Medicine, Rome, Italy

A. Frund   Heart and Diabetes Center, Department of Physiotherapy, Bad Oeynhausen, North Rhine-Westphalia, Germany

Barbara Di Giacinto, MD   Institute of Sport Medicine and Science, Italian National Olympic Committee, Department of Sport Medicine, Rome, Italy, barbara.digiacinto@virgilio.it

Emanuele Guerra, MD Institute of Sport Medicine and Science, Italian National Olympic Committee, Department of Sport Medicine, Rome, Italy, casaguerra@alice.it

Terje Halvorsen, MD Norwegian institute of Sports Medicine, Oslo, Norway

Finn Hegbom, MD, PhD Center for Arrhythmia, Oslo, Norway

Giancarlo Magri, MD Department of Nuclear Medicine, Spedali Civili, Brescia, Italy

K.-P. Mellwig, MD Department of Sports Cardiology, Bad Oeynhausen, North Rhine-Westphalia, Germany

Peter Mills, MA, BSc, FRCP Department of Cardiology, The London Chest Hospital, London, England

E. Oepangat, MD Heart and Diabetes Centre, Department of Cardiology, Bad Oeynhausen, North Rhine–Westphalia, Germany

O. Oldenburg, MD Heart and Diabetes Centre, Department of Cardiology, Bad Oeynhausen, North Rhine–Westphalia, Germany

Fernando Maria Di Paolo, MD Institute of Sport Medicine and Science, Italian National Olympic Committee, Department of Medicine, Rome, Italy, fernando.dipaolo@guest.coni.it

Evasio Pasini, MD Department of Cardiology, Fondazione S. Maugeri, Lumezzane, Brescia, Italy

Camille Pesch, MD Hospital Centre of Luxembourg, Department of Cardiology, Luxembourg

Cataldo Pisicchio, MD Institute of Sport Medicine and Science, Italian National Olympic Committee, Department of Medicine, Rome, Italy, aldopis@gmail.com

Filippo M. Quattrini, MD, PhD Institute of Sport Medicine and Science, Italian National Olympic Committee, Department of Medicine, Rome, Italy, f.quattrini@guest.coni.it

John Rawlins, BSc, MRCP Department of Cardiology, King's College Hospital, London

Sanjay Sharma, BSc (Hons), MB ChB, MD, FRCP (UK), FESC Department of Cardiology, King's College Hospital, Denmark Hill, London, UK, ssharma21@hotmail.com

Nadir Sitta, MD Cardiology Unit, Conegliano Hospital, Conegliano, Italy

Joep L.R.M. Smeets, MD, PhD Department of Cardiology, University Medical Center, Radboud University, Nijmegen, The Netherlands

Erik Ekker Solberg, MD, PhD, FESC Diakonhjemmet Hospital, Medical Department, 0319 Oslo, Norway, erik.solberg@diakonsyk.no

Knut-Haakon Stensaeth, MD Department of Cardiovascular Radiology, Ulleval University Hospital, Oslo, Norway

Mohamed Tahmi, MD, PhD Department of Cardiology, CHU Tizi Ouzou, Nedir Hospital-Tizi-Ouzou University, Tizi Ouzou, Algeria, mtahmi@hotmail.com

A.W. Treusch, MD Department of Cardiology, Leopoldina Hospital, Schweinfurt, Germany, atreush@hdz-nrw.de

Axel J.P. Urhausen, MD, PhD Service de Medecine du Sport et de Prevention, Centre de l' Appareil Locomoteur, de Medecine du Sport et de Prevention, Centre, Hospitalier de Luxembourg-Clinique d'Eich, Luxembourg, urhausen.axel@chl.lu

Luisa Verdile, MD Institute of Sports Medicine and Science, Italian National Olympic Committee, Department of Medicine, Rome, Italy, luisa.verdile@coni.it

Introduction

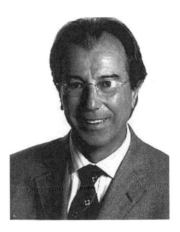

Over recent years, issues related to management of competitive and amateur athletes with cardiovascular disease have (CV) become highly visible and complex medical and public health topics. Particular interest surrounds these issues in consideration that elite and professional athletes represent a special and visible subset of our society, not only for their outstanding physical performances, but also for the substantial economic interests and the intense pressure to which they are exposed by sponsors, sports organizations and media [1–4].

When a cardiovascular disease is found in such athletes, the managing physician is required to solve the compelling issue of appropriate management and recommendations, considering both the impact of sport participation on the course and outcome of cardiac disease and the impact of disqualification on the athlete's life.

In the last 2 decades participation in a broad spectrum of sport activities (including competitive events) has increased substantially in civilized societies and has become an integral part of the lifestyle of large segments of the population, including very young and senior individuals. In this context, competitive and professional sports have progressively evolved toward globalization, including nowadays not only Western Europe and the U.S., but also large number of East European and African countries, as evident by the changing demographics of elite athletes engaged in professional sports, primarily soccer or basketball.

Due to the unique structure and pressures of competitive sports, athletes with CV disease may not always have adequate knowledge and independent judgment in assessing the risk associated with a competitive sports career. Therefore, the managing physician (and consultant cardiologist) have the ethical, medical and legal obligation to assess appropriately the overall risk scenario associated with sport lifestyle in an athlete with cardiovascular abnormality and clearly inform the candidate. Indeed, the managing physician is responsible for final recommendations concerning sport participation, with the aim to preserve the innumerable benefits derived from sport (including economic interests in elite/professional athletes) but prevent adverse clinical events and reduce the risk of disease progression.

However, when a disqualification decision is possible, pressure on the managing physician may be intense, and consensus guidelines represent the only legitimate support to the physician's decision. Under such difficult circumstances, adherence to recommendations released by scientific societies represents the only appropriate defense for the physician, as well as the appropriate manner in which to protect athletes from the unsustainable hazard of sports participation.

Consensus guidelines for eligibility/disqualification decisions in competitive athletes with cardiovascular abnormalities were initially promoted in the U.S. (in 1985 the American College of Cardiology formalized the first Bethesda Conference #16, with subsequent updated #26 and #36 in 1994 and 2005, respectively [5–7]). In Europe, the first consensus document concerning the management and participation in competitive sports of athletes with cardiovascular abnormalities was delivered from the Italian Sports Cardiology Society in 1995 and subsequently updated to 2003 [8], and from the European Society of Cardiology (ESC) in 2005 [9].

The rationale for offering both the American and European expert consensus documents is the widely accepted perception that athletes with clinically silent cardiovascular disease harbor increased risk for disease progression and sudden death by virtue of their commitment to intensive training and competition. Conversely, the removal of athletes from this lifestyle is regarded as mechanism by which the risk may be substantially reduced [10, 11].

Both the ACC Bethesda Conference #36 and the ESC recommendations provide specific advice with respect to different cardiac abnormalities and sports, based on the available scientific data, as well as on personal experience of the panel participants. These documents represent the most updated attempt to combine the (scarce) evidence-based data with personal experience of the experts.

However, presentation of cardiovascular disease in individual athletes may present a variety of clinical forms and not always correspond to the schemes reported in the documents, making management of the candidate-athlete troublesome. In these instances it is challenging to translate the recommendations dictated by the scientific societies into the clinical practice.

It was our aim to address this problem with the present textbook entitled "Sports Cardiology Casebook". It was our intention to provide the managing physician with appropriate tools for solving this problem, i.e., examples derived from the clinical practice, which illustrate how to proceed in the management and final recommendations of an athlete with cardiovascular abnormality by applying the current consensus guidelines.

The textbook includes a large selection of clinical cases, which are intended to offer a wide perspective of the most common problems arising in the cardiovascular evaluation of competitive athletes, as viewed by expert European cardiologists. The selected cases are listed according to their clinical presentations, i.e., abnormalities discovered by medical history, by the electrocardiogram, and finally by the usual imaging testing (primarily, echocardiography). This structure makes it easy for the physician to search for a similar and appropriate tutorial case.

The clinical cases here reported represent the selection made by physicians and scientists working in Europe within the Sports Cardiology group, and their assessment closely reflect the ESC consensus guidelines [9], in addition to their personal expertise and science. However, in consideration of the scarcity of scientific investigations concerning the effect of regular sport activities on the pathophysiology and clinical course of several cardiovascular disease, caution is needed in applying the present examples to clinical practice, and efforts should be made to tailor precise advice to each athlete-patient.

Therefore, the examples provided here cannot be assumed to represent the standard of care in all instances, but are examples to be applied in practice in a individualized fashion. Indeed, these cases should not restrict the physician's independent judgment in evaluating the candidate-athlete and cannot be claimed as impairment to physician liberty to search appropriately the best medical management of the patient-athlete.

References

1. Maron BJ. Sudden death in young athletes: lessons from the Hank Gathers affair. N Engl J Med 1993, 329:55–57
2. Maron BJ, Mitten MJ, Quandt EK, et al. Competitive athletes with cardiovascular disease: the case of Nicholas Knapp. N Engl J Med 1998, 339:1623–1625
3. Maron BJ. Sudden death in young athletes. New Engl J Med 2003, 349: 1064–1075
4. Thompson PD, Franklin BA, Balady G, Blair SN, Corrado D, Mark Estes NA III, Fulton JE, Gordon NF, Haskell WL, Link MS, Maron BJ, Mittleman MA, Pelliccia A, Wenger NK, Willich SN, Costa F. Exercise and acute cardiovascular events: placing the risks into perspective. Scientific Statement from the American Heart Association Council on Nutrition, Physical Activity, and Metabolism and the Council on Clinical Cardiology. In collaboration with the American College of Sports Medicine. Circulation 2007, 115:2358–2368
5. Mitchell JH, Maron BJ, Epstein SE. 16th Bethesda Conference: cardiovascular abnormalities in the athlete: recommendations regarding eligibility for competition. J Am Coll Cardiol 1985, 6:1186–1232
6. Maron BJ, Mitchell JH. 26th Bethesda Conference: cardiovascular abnormalities: recommendations for determining eligibility for competition in athletes with cardiovascular abnormalities. J Am Coll Cardiol 1994, 24:845–899
7. Maron, BJ, Zipes DP. 36th Bethesda Conference: Eligibility recommendations for competitive athletes with cardiovascular abnormalities. J Am Coll Cardiol 2005, 45:2–64.
8. Comitato organizzativo cardiologico per l'idoneità allo sport. Protocolli cardiologici per il giudizio di idoneità allo sport agonistico 2003. Med Sport 2004, 57:375–438
9. Pelliccia A, Fagard R, Bjørnstad HH, Anastassakis A, Arbustini E, Assanelli D, Biffi A, Borjesson M, Carrè F, Corrado D, Delise P, Dorwarth U, Hirth A, Heidbuchel H, Hoffmann E, Mellwig KP, Panhuyzen-Goedkoop N, Pisani A, Solberg E, van-Buuren F, Vanhees L. Recommendations for competitive sports participation in athletes with cardiovascular disease. A consensus document from the Study Group of Sports Cardiology of the Working Group of Cardiac Rehabilitation and Exercise Physiology, and the Working Group of Myocardial and Pericardial diseases of the European Society of Cardiology. Eur Heart J 2005, 26:1422–1445

10. Corrado D, Basso C, Rizzoli G, Schiavon M, Thiene G. Does sport activity enhance the risk of sudden death in adolescents and young adults? J Am Coll Cardiol 2003, 42:1959–1963
11. Biffi A, Maron BJ, Verdile L, Fernando F, Spataro A, Marcello G, Ciardo R, Ammirati F, Colivicchi F, Pelliccia A. Impact of physical deconditioning on ventricular tachyarrhythmias in trained athletes. J Am Coll Cardiol 2004, 44:1053–1058

Chapter 1
A 27-Year-Old Professional Cyclist with Palpitations on Effort

Hein Heidbüchel and Axel J.P. Urhausen

Family and Personal History

The patient was a 27-year-old professional cyclist. An elite athlete, he had partic-ipated at several international races, including the *Tour the France* and the World Cycling Championship.

Prior medical history was uneventful. There were no familial antecedents of sud-den cardiac death. His father and younger brother were competitive cyclists too, albeit not at a professional level.

The athlete was referred to our observation because of recurrent exercised-induced palpitations that had first occurred 1 month before.

The athlete reported that during exercise the heart rate monitor showed abrupt increase of heart rate, from an average of 170–180 bpm, to 210 bpm for a few sec-onds. At that moment the athlete experienced palpitations and a sudden fatigue, but no dizziness. He never had a pre-syncope or syncope. It was remarkable that the team physician had, because of these palpitations, given him flecainide IV on the morning before a competition, although no prior ECG diagnosis had been made. Apparently the treatment had been successful in preventing recurrences.

Physical Examination

The physical examination was normal. Blood pressure was 124/72 mmHg.

12-Lead ECG

The ECG at first evaluation is shown in Fig. 1.1. There was a sinus rate of 42 bpm. The QRS complex duration was slightly prolonged (105 ms) with mild,

H. Heidbüchel (✉)
Department of Cardiology, University Hospital Gasthuisberg, University of Leuven, Herestraat 49
B-3000 Leuven, Belgium, Europe
e-mail: Hein.Heidbuchel@uz.kuleuven.ac.be

A. Pelliccia (ed.), *Sports Cardiology Casebook*,
DOI 10.1007/978-1-84882-042-5_1, © Springer-Verlag London Limited 2009

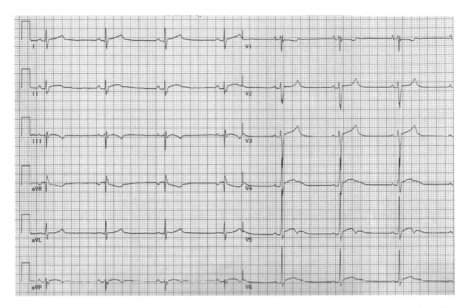

Fig. 1.1 The 12-lead ECG at initial evaluation. There was a sinus rate of 42 bpm. The QRS complex was slightly prolonged (105 ms) with a QTc interval of 520 ms. and repolarization abnormalities (the QTc interval was normal on an ECG 2 years earlier, and there were no indications for familial long QT syndrome)

non-specific repolarization changes. The corrected QTc interval was markedly prolonged (520 ms).

A prior ECG was searched for (recorded during a cardiologic screening performed elsewhere 2 years before): at that time the ECG showed a QTc interval within normal limits (i.e., 440 ms).

Diagnostic Testing

The exercise test showed a superb performance, with maximum workload of 550 W and heart rate of 180 bpm. During the test, the QTc interval returned to normal limits (<440 ms), but there was a progressive widening of the QRS complex, with development of a right bundle branch block morphology and indeterminate axis (Figs. 1.2 and 1.3 at 200 W and 500 W workloads, respectively). During the recovery the QRS width decreased gradually.

In addition, sporadic premature ventricular beats (PVBs) with different morphology (mostly with left bundle branch block) were observed during exercise.

The ECG Holter monitoring documented 870 PVBs/24 h, with different morphology.

A late potential ECG was positive for three criteria (filtered QRS duration 139 ms; HFLA duration 56 ms and RMS40 17 μV; Fig. 1.4).

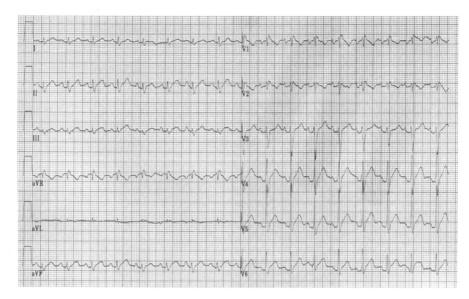

Fig. 1.2 The ECG recorded at 200 W during exercise testing. There is sinus tachycardia with a rate of 100 bpm. Compared to the baseline ECG, there is a shortening of the QTc interval, but a slight increase of the QRS duration with an incomplete right bundle branch pattern is seen

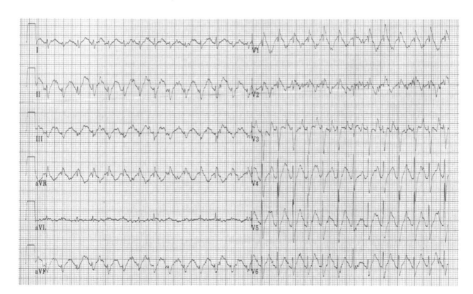

Fig. 1.3 The ECG recorded at 500 W during exercise testing. There is a further increase of the QRS duration with development of complete right bundle branch block

Fig. 1.4 Late potentials were present with three out of three positive criteria: filtered QRS duration 139 ms (normal ≤120 ms); duration of the high-frequency low-amplitude signals ≤40 μV (HFLA40) 56 ms (normal <40 ms), and root mean square voltage of the last 40 ms (RMS40) 17 μV (normal >20 μV)

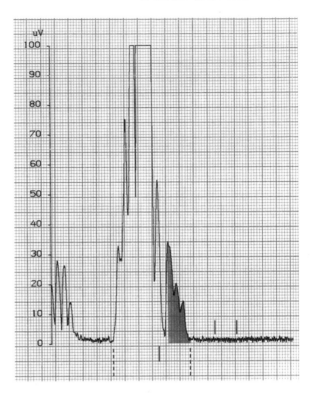

Echocardiography showed dilatation of the left ventricle (diastolic and systolic diameter 58 mm and 38 mm, respectively) with concordant dilatation of the other heart chambers. LV septal thickness was 15 mm and posterior wall thickness 12 mm. The overall morphologic pattern was judged to be expression of the athlete's heart [1].

Cardiac magnetic resonance imaging excluded hypertrophic cardiomyopathy, but showed a disproportionate (albeit mild) dilatation of the right ventricle (RV) with slightly reduced systolic function. Early diastolic flattening of the septum and a distended inferior vena cava suggested RV overload.

Coronary angiography and ventriculography showed normal coronary arteries, a slightly dilated but normally contractile left ventricle, and a slightly dilated and mildly hypokinetic right ventricle, without significant regional wall motion abnormalities.

An electrophysiological (EP) study was performed. It excluded a concealed accessory pathway and AV nodal re-entrant tachycardia. It could not induce any atrial arrhythmias nor any ventricular arrhythmias (with up to three extra stimuli at two basic cycle lengths of 600 and 400 ms at baseline, and after administration of 1, 2 and 3 μg/min of isoprenaline). During isoprenaline infusion, however, sporadic PVBs and couplets, again with left bundle branch morphology and variable axis, were induced.

In conclusion, the cardiovascular evaluation suggested abnormal ventricular conduction slowing throughout the ventricles, of unknown aetiology, associated with
PVBs and positive late potentials. Moreover, there were signs of RV overload (which
were likely related to the frequent PVBs with left bundle branch morphology), but
these abnormalities did not fulfil the criteria for arrhythmogenic RV cardiomyopathy (ARVC). Together with the late potentials, there were two minor criteria for
ARVC, which were not sufficient for definite diagnosis [2].

Recommendations and Treatment

The patient was advised to stop competitive sports and was requested to perform
only moderate training with a long-term ECG recorder and his rate monitor, with
the purpose of recording the spontaneous arrhythmias.

Two weeks later an event recording during training revealed polymorphic ventricular tachycardia which lasted more than 15 s. It reproduced the subjective symptoms and was recorded as an abrupt heart rate acceleration on his heart rate monitor
(Fig. 1.5).

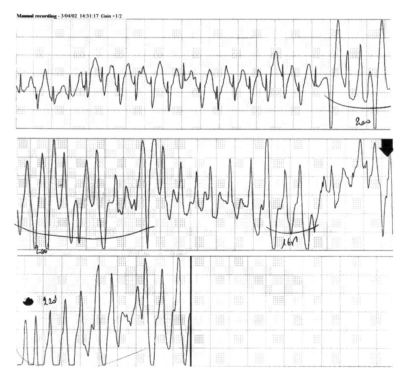

Fig. 1.5 Event recording during training revealing polymorphic ventricular tachycardia which
lasted >15 s. It reproduced the subjective symptoms and was documented as an heart rate acceleration on his heart rate monitor

Clinical Course

The athlete was advised to stop any competitive and intensive sports activity. A low dose beta-blocker was started (metoprolol 25 mg once daily). Class-1 drugs or amiodarone were considered to be an unsuitable option given the intraventricular conduction delays. It was also suggested to consider prophylactic ICD implantation, which the athlete declined.

Given the impact of the therapeutic decisions, the athlete was advised to seek a second opinion. The importance of showing all the available data for such a second opinion was stressed, and a file with copied documents was assembled for this purpose.

The patient consulted six other cardiology centers, taking the documentation of the original evaluation with him. In four the same advice was given, whereas in two others the recommendation was given to continue competitive sports under beta-blocker treatment, based on the finding that arrhythmias during exercise tests were non inducible under treatment with metoprolol 25 mg/day. The patient, therefore, restarted competition.

Nevertheless, 6 months later and despite continued beta-blocker treatment the athlete showed an exercised-induced non-sustained ventricular tachycardia (10 beats, 220 bpm) during exercise testing performed in one of the latter centers. At that time, also in that center the athlete was finally advised to stop any competitive sports activity.

After 1 year he was admitted to yet another hospital with sustained ventricular tachycardia which had developed during recreational cycling (230/min.). A new EP study was performed, which triggered two sustained ventricular tachycardias, both with left bundle branch block morphology. An ICD was recommended, but rejected again by the patient.

After 6 months he was re-admitted to yet another hospital with sustained ventricular tachycardia (the trigger of which is unknown). Ablation was not performed since it was not considered to be definitive treatment. An ICD was recommended based on the evidence of progressive arrhythmogenic disease in the athlete, albeit without unequivocal diagnosis of ARVC. The patient again rejected the ICD.

After 2 months he collapsed during a solo cycling training, was resuscitated late and died 2 weeks later.

Discussion

This case illustrates the difficult work-up of an athlete presenting with palpitations, and the difficulty in coming to a conclusive diagnosis on the aetiology of ventricular arrhythmias, which may convey a lethal outcome.

It also illustrates the special care needed in evaluating athletes with palpitations induced by exercise, such as in this case, where ventricular conduction disturbances and right ventricular enlargement were seen, but it was unclear whether the palpitations were due to repetitive ventricular premature beats or ventricular tachyarrhythmia or sustained atrial arrhythmia.

Imaging examinations are not always sufficient for diagnosis, as in this case, where the electrophysiological work-up was warranted. Indeed, although the initial QTc interval in our patient was prolonged, there was no further evidence for a congenital long QT syndrome (which was also excluded by the familial screening). This case is also certainly not a typical presentation of catecholaminergic polymorphic VT and there was no familial history of it.

On the other hand, there was conduction abnormality (right bundle branch block; late potentials), increasing during faster heart rates, and of progressive nature.

Some authors have suggested that, in the absence of epsilon-waves on the surface-ECG, signal-averaged ECG recording revealing late potentials may be a sign of delayed (right) ventricular activation and of a pro-arrhythmogenic substrate [3]. Late potentials may be a subtle but definite criterion for ARVC [2]. Unfortunately, genotyping was not available to exclude further a channelopathy or cardiomyopathy in this case. Eventually, not only the absence of a familial history but also the progressive nature of the conduction disturbances (with a normal ECG pattern seen 2 years before presentation) argues against pre-existing and/or familial disease.

Polymorphic ventricular tachycardia occurring during exercise, as documented in this case, always carries a bad prognosis, since it may point to an underlying inherited electrophysiological disorder or to underlying structural disease.

Given the undeniable presence of underlying pathologic substrate (albeit without conclusive diagnosis), this patient was definitely considered ineligible for competitive sports like cycling [4]. Although this advise was debated after the first evaluation, there was clear medical consent in this respect after documentation of repeat arrhythmias, despite beta-blocker treatment.

A sense of concern is also related to the inability for the several consultant cardiologists to implement their advise into practice. The lack of national law obliging athletes to obtain a medical clearance before entering competitive sport (such is the case in Italy) put the cardiologists in the position of not being able to withdraw this patient at high risk from sport activity.

In conclusion, palpitations during exercise, fast rates on a heart rate monitor, symptoms of hemodynamic compromise (like a sudden fatigue during exercise in this case), and even the finding of sporadic VPBs during an exercise test should be taken seriously and should trigger a comprehensive evaluation for ruling out underlying structural heart disease and potentially lethal ventricular tachyarrhythmia (see also Chapters 19 and 21 in this respect).

That goal needs a tailored and individualised work-up in selected cases, and may also exceed the standard routine protocol suggested in the recommendations [4].

References

1. Maron BJ, Pellicia A. The heart of trained athletes: cardiac remodeling and the risks of sports, including sudden death. Circulation 2006, 10(114):1633–1644
2. McKenna WJ, Thiene G, Nava A, Fontaliran F, Blomstrom Lundqvist C, Fontaine G, Camerini F. Diagnosis of arrhythmogenic right ventricular dysplasia/cardiomyopathy. Task Force of the Working Group Myocardial and Pericardial Disease of the European Society of

Cardiology and of the Scientific Council on Cardiomyopathies of the International Society and Federation of Cardiology. Br Heart J 1994, 71(3):215–218

3. Jordaens L, Missault L, Pelleman G, Duprez D, De Backer G, Clement DL. Comparison of athletes with life-threatening ventricular arrhythmias with two groups of healthy athletes and a group of normal control subjects. Am J Cardiol 1994, 74(11):1124–1128

4. Heidbuchel H, Corrado D, Biffi A, Hoffmann E, Panhuyzen-Goedkoop N, Hoogsteen J, Delise P, Hoff PI, Pelliccia A. Recommendations for participation in leisure-time physical activity and competitive sports of patients with arrhythmias and potentially arrhythmogenic conditions. Part II: Ventricular arrhythmias, channelopathies and implantable defibrillators. Eur J Cardiovasc Prev Rehabil Oct 2006, 13(5):676–686

Chapter 2
Impaired Performance in a Master Long-Distance Runner

François Carré

History

A 58-year-old male long distance runner complained of reduced exertion performance during the last 3 months despite an intensive training schedule. He felt "broken" beyond 12 km/h, and experienced respiratory "blockage" during high speed running, associated with a dramatic decrease of his maximal running speed. During the last 5 years he had short episodes of palpitations during training. Previous cardiovascular testing (12-leads ECG, echocardiography, maximal exercise test, ECG Holter monitoring) demonstrated a few isolated supraventricular and ventricular premature beats. His general physician recently performed a comprehensive haematological check-up, which showed no abnormalities.

Athletic History

This athlete has been active in long distance running for the last 20 years and participated in long-distance events, from half-marathon to 100-km races. The current training schedule was between 80 and 100 km per week (five sessions a week of running and one session of cycling).

Family History

His familial history revealed no known congenital or other cardiovascular diseases and no known cases of premature (< 50 years) sudden cardiac death in close relatives.

F. Carré (✉)
Department of Physiology, Unité de Biologie.et de Médecine du Sport, Pontchaillou Hospital*,*.
Rennes 1 University, INSERM U 642, France
e-mail: francois.carre@univ-rennes1.fr

A. Pelliccia (ed.), *Sports Cardiology Casebook*,
DOI 10.1007/978-1-84882-042-5_2, © Springer-Verlag London Limited 2009

Medication

He does not use any medication, and denies any drugs abuse.

Physical Examination

On physical examination there was a healthy male, height 1.69 m, weight 66 kg, with a calculated fat mass of 19%. His resting heart rate was 48 bpm, and blood pressure 145/90 mmHg. Auscultation of heart and lungs was normal.

12-Lead ECG

Resting 12-lead ECG (Fig. 2.1) shows a sinus bradycardia (45 bpm). The PR, QRS, and QT/QTc intervals were normal. The P wave was somewhat enlarged and split in standard leads, negative in standard lead III, in precordial lead V1 and diphasic in V2. An incomplete right bundle branch block was noted. Flat and negative T waves were present in precordial leads from V4 to V6. One isolated ventricular premature beat was registered.

All these ECG changes were already noted in previous ECG tracings and the present pattern had remained substantially unchanged over the last few years.

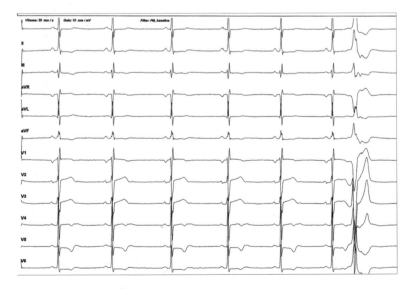

Fig. 2.1 Resting 12-lead ECG pattern

Maximal Exercise Test with Gas Analysis

Because of the symptoms, runner's age and resting ECG changes, we performed maximal exercise test with gas analysis. The test was performed on a treadmill and was interrupted at the occurrence of dyspnoea and subjective feeling of respiratory "blockage". The athlete reached the maximum speed of 12.5 km/h, which was maintained for only 2 min. Maximal heart rate was 144 bpm. Gas analysis showed a maximal oxygen uptake of 3 L/min (43 mL/min/kg) which represent 130% of the theoretical value (Fig. 2.1).

Because of the runner's training level, a higher performance was expected, and the present performance was decreased in comparison to exercise testing of the previous year, which showed maximal speed of 14.5 km/h at the same maximal heart rate attained (143 bpm). Moreover, the behaviour of oxygen pulse showed an early plateau with a significant decrease before the end of the test (Fig. 2.1). This pattern was consistent with a decreasing stroke volume. The ECG showed a straight downward ST-segment in precordial lead V6 (Fig. 2.1), which quickly disappeared during the recovery. Unfortunately blood pressure was not measured during the treadmill test.

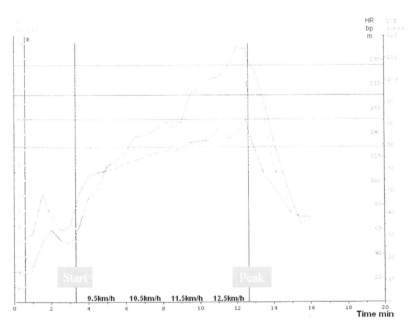

Fig. 2.2 Maximal exercise with expired gas analysis on treadmill. A progressive continuous protocol with a constant 1% slope grade and a 1 km/h increase every 2 min was used. $V'O_2 = O_2$ uptake, $V'CO_2 = CO_2$ production, $V'E$ = ventilation; HR = heart rate

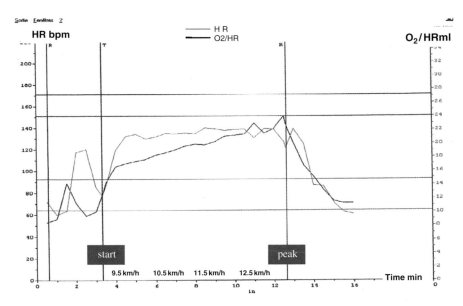

Fig. 2.3 Maximal exercise with expired gas analysis on treadmill. A progressive continuous protocol with a constant 1% slope grade and a 1 km/h increase every 2 min was used. HR = heart rate; V'O$_2$/HR = O$_2$ pulse

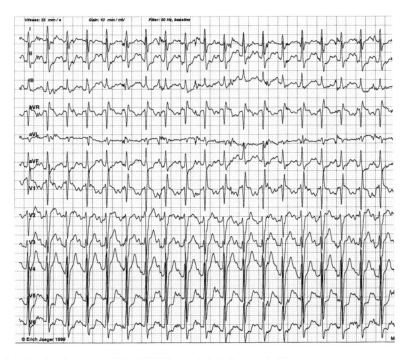

Fig. 2.4 Maximal exercise 12-lead ECG recorded during treadmill test

Trans-Thoracic Echocardiography

Resting echocardiography showed end-diastolic LV diameter of 54 mm, with ventricular septum and posterior free wall thickness at the upper normal limits (11–12 mm). Left atrium (transverse diameter, 49 mm) was dilated. Systolic function (ejection fraction: 62%) and mitral filling pattern were normal. A mild mitral insufficiency and a mild tricuspid insufficiency (grade I, pulmonary arterial pressure 18 mmHg) were noted.

Stress Echocardiography

Physical stress was performed on a bicycle exercise in semi-supine position. Maximal power was 200 W, with a maximum heart rate of 135 bpm. Maximal blood pressure was abnormally increased, i.e., 255/118 mmHg and decreased slowly to 164/86 mmHg after 6 min of recovery, at heart rate 65 bpm. No significant arrhythmia were observed. Repolarization showed the same patterns as observed during the treadmill test, i.e., straight downward ST-segment in precordial leads.

Echocardiography on peak exertion revealed no segmental wall motion abnormalities and ejection fraction of 80%, but a substantially increased pulmonary artery pressure of 45 mmHg.

Diagnosis and Recommendations

Based on these results, diagnosis of systemic hypertension was made, based on the consideration that resting blood pressure (145/90 mmHg) was somewhat too high for a well trained long-distance runner. Moreover, blood pressure was substantially increased at peak exercise, in consideration of the workload performed. Lastly, left atrium was increased. The marked increase of the after-load during strenuous exercise due to underlying systemic hypertension was believed to explain the drop in oxygen pulse observed and the shortness of breath described by the runner. We recommended an ACE inhibitor and refrained the athlete from competitions until blood pressure control was achieved. Treatment was efficient to decrease blood pressure and relieve symptoms. At follow-up (after 12 months) the athlete was asymptomatic and blood pressure was normal at rest (140/85 mmHg) and on maximum exertion (230 W, BP 210/80 mmHg, HR 142 bpm). He was eligible for competitive sports without limitations and his performance is similar to that achieved in previous years.

Discussion

This 58-year-old male endurance athlete suffered from symptomatic hypertension at rest and on exertion. Limitation of exercise tolerance and shortness of breath on exertion were the first symptoms.

When an athlete shows borderline blood pressure at rest, it is of utmost importance to measure the blood pressure on exertion and to assess the overall risk profile. Advice regarding participation in sports activity is, in fact, based on the global risk profile, which also include blood pressure. According to the recommendations [1,2], β-blockers and diuretics should not be the first choice of treatment in an athlete with hypertension, but ACE inhibitors, angiotensin II antagonists and calcium channel blockers should be preferred.

References

1. Pelliccia A, Fagard R, Bjørnstad HH, Anastassakis A, Arbustini E, Assanelli D, Biffi A, Borjesson M, Carrè F, Corrado D, Delise P, Dorwarth U, Hirth A,. Heidbuchel H, Hoffmann E, Mellwig KP, Panhuyzen-Goedkoop N, Pisani A, Solberg E, van-Buuren F, Vanhees L. Recommendations for competitive sports participation in athletes with cardiovascular disease. A consensus document from the Study Group of Sports Cardiology of the Working Group of Cardiac Rehabilitation and Exercise Physiology, and the Working Group of Myocardial and Pericardial diseases of the European Society of Cardiology. Eur Heart J 2005, 26:1422–1445
2. Fagard RH, Bjørnstad HH, Borjesson M, Carrè F, Deligiannis A, Vanhees L. ESC study group of sports cardiology recommendations for participation in leisure-time physical activities and competitive sports for patients with hypertension. Eur J Prev Cardiovasc Rehabil 2005, 12: 326–331

Chapter 3
A 26-Year-Old Cyclist with Syncope on Effort

Nicole M. Panhuyzen-Goedkoop and Joep L.R.M. Smeets

Family and Personal History

This is a 26-year-old male, with no known congenital or other cardiovascular disease in the family. No known cases of premature (<50 years) sudden cardiac death among close relatives.

The patient was actively engaged in top-level professional cycling, and achieved an international level of recognition. His training schedule included 5 6 sessions a week, 2 5 hours(h) of cycling indoor and outdoor (cross training and on the road).

Medical History

This young male occasionally suffered from dizziness and lightheadedness during indoor training. After stepping down from the bike, and sitting down in a squat position, complaints disappeared in a few minutes, and he could resume training without further problems. For this reason he was referred to elsewhere for consultation.

Physical Examination

On physical examination blood pressure was normal, 110/60 mmHg, and there were no cardiac murmurs or abnormal heart sounds.

12-Lead ECG

On the 12-lead resting ECG there was sinus rhythm, normal QRS axis, normal AV conduction. The R/S wave voltages in precordial leads were increased, compatible

N.M. Panhuyzen-Goedkoop (✉)
Department of Sports Cardiology, Sint Maartenskliniek, Location Sports Medical Centre Papendal, Radboud University Hospital Nijmegen, Arnhem, The Netherlands
e-mail: n.panhuyzen@smcp.nl

A. Pelliccia (ed.), *Sports Cardiology Casebook*,
DOI 10.1007/978-1-84882-042-5_3, © Springer-Verlag London Limited 2009

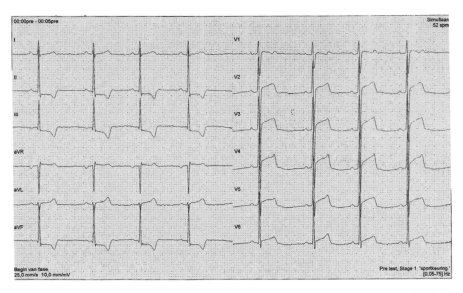

Fig. 3.1 Baseline 12-lead ECG of the athlete. Increased R/S wave voltages in precordial leads (V2–V6) are evident, in association with abnormal repolarization pattern (depressed ST segment, inverted T waves) in standard leads II, III, aVF

with LV hypertrophy and marked abnormal ST-T wave changes were evident in standard leads II, III and aVF (Fig. 3.1).

Echocardiography

Echocardiographic findings were within normal limits (Table 3.1). Although the LV posterior free wall was at upper normal limits, there was no evidence of segmental hypertrophy and the overall picture was suggestive for physiologic cardiac

Table 3.1 Cardiac dimension of the patient as assesses by echocardiography

Cardiac structure	Cardiac dimensions	Normal values in cyclists (according to [11])
LVDd	56 mm	58±4 mm
VS	10 mm	≤12 mm
PW	12 mm	≤12 mm
Doppler-derived velocity		
Ao Vmax	1.36 m/s	1.0–1.7 m/s
PV Vmax	0.80 m/s	0.6–0.9 m/s
E/A ratio	2.0	1.9±0.6

LVDd = Left ventricular diastolic diameter; VS = Ventricular septal thickness; PW = Posterior; Ao = aortic valve; PV = pulmonary valve; E/A ratio = ratio of the early diastolic to late diastolic peak flow velocities assessed at level mitral valve

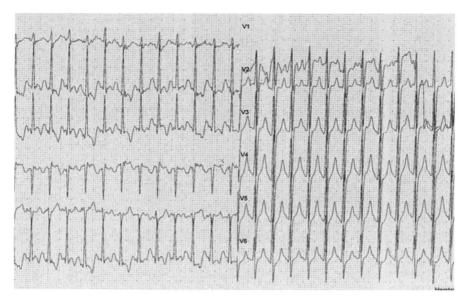

Fig. 3.2 Electrocardiogram recorded during exercise testing. Note the T wave alternans in the standard inferior leads

remodeling, and not for hypertrophic cardiomyopathy. Left ventricular function was normal and so was the diastolic filling pattern, as assessed by transmitral Doppler echocardiography. No abnormalities were found regarding right ventricular morphology and function.

Exercise Electrocardiography

On exercise testing, starting from 75 W for 4 min, with increments of 50 W every 1 min, he reached 400 W, with a maximal heart rate of 185 bpm, and showed a normal increment of the blood pressure (at rest 135/75 mmHg, at peak exertion 240/95 mmHg). There were no symptoms and no premature ventricular beats (PVBs) or other arrhythmia during exertion. However, during exercise test T-wave alternans was present in the standard inferior leads (Fig. 3.2).

Despite the abnormal ECG pattern, and in consideration of the absence of cardiac structural alterations detectable by echocardiography, the patient was cleared for competition.

Clinical Course

Two months later he had a sub-febrile temperature for 2 days, and an increased resting heart rate of 15–20 bpm (resting heart rate, from the usual 40 to 55–60 bpm) for 4 days. On the 5th day his resting heart rate returned to usual value, and on the

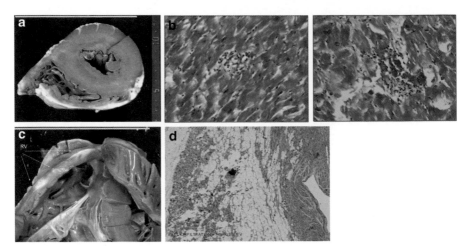

Fig. 3.3a–d Cardiac pathology findings in the athlete. **a,b** Left ventricle with diffuse inflammatory spots. **c,d** Right ventricle with diffuse fatty infiltration and fibrosis (with permission of AC van der Wal, Acad Med Center. Amsterdam)

same day he resumed training. On the 7th day, after 1 h from his training session, without any premonitory symptoms, he suddenly collapsed while driving home and lost consciousness. His friends almost immediately started resuscitation, without success.

The autopsy assessment revealed heart weight increased (700 g), left ventricle with diffuse transmural inflammatory spots (leukocyte infiltration with necrosis and myocyte degeneration), and right ventricle with diffuse fatty infiltration and fibrosis (Fig. 3.3). This pattern was judged consistent with the diagnosis of arrhythmogenic right ventricular cardiomyopathy (ARVC) [1]. Diagnosis was confirmed by a second opinion elsewhere. DNA analysis was performed but did not reveal any of the reported gene abnormalities associated with ARVC, such as PKP2, DSP desmoplakin on chromosome 6p24, DSG2 desmoglycin on chromosome 18q12.1-q12.2, RyR2 ryanodine receptor, or DSC2 on chromosome 18q12.1 [2, 3].

In conclusion, final diagnosis in this 26-year-old top-level cyclist who suffered from exercise induced syncope was, based on autopsy finding, arrhythmogenic right ventricular cardiomyopathy.

Discussion

Syncope (or pre-syncope) during exertion in young athletes is an alarming symptom, and first clinical expression of cardiomyopathies (HCM, ARVC), channelopaties, myocarditis, valvular/subvalvular disease, high-grade AV block, congenital coronary anomaly or critical coronary artery disease [4]. Pathology findings in this case demonstrated ARVC with inflammatory spots in the ventricles.

Table 3.2 Current major and minor criteria for diagnosis of ARVC

Major criteria
Familial disease confirmed at necropsy or surgery
Epsilon wave or QRS duration >110 ms in V1-V3
Severe RV dilatation and systolic dysfunction with no/mild LV involvement
Localized RV aneurysms (akinetic/dyskinetic areas with diastolic bulgings)
Severe segmental RV dilatation
Fibrofatty replacement of myocardium (endomyocardial biopsy)

Minor criteria
Family history of premature sudden death (<35 years)
Family history based on clinical diagnostic criteria
Late potentials (signal-averaged ECG)
Inverted T waves in V2 and V3, no RBBB, in patients >12 years
LBBB-type tachycardia (sustained or non-sustained) on ECG, Holter monitoring or during
    exercise testing
Ventricular extrasystoles (>1000 in 24 h) on Holter monitoring
Mild global reduced RV dilatation and/or RV dysfunction with preserved LV function
Mild segmental RV dilatation
Regional RV wall motion

According to the current clinical practice two major criteria, or one major and two minor criteria are necessary for the diagnosis of ARVC (Table 3.2) [5, 6]. In most instances, however, such as was the case of this athlete, definite diagnosis cannot be reached according to these criteria. In fact, in our athlete the most typical electrocardiographic changes (inverted T waves in anterior precordial leads, or right ventricular conduction delays, or epsilon wave, or ventricular ectopic beats with LBBB morphology) were absent. Indeed, the echocardiographic investigation failed to show any global or segmental morphologic alteration in the right ventricle. These findings suggest the need for revising diagnostic criteria for this disease and that great clinical expertise and caution is due in diagnosis of ARVC. Most young patients with ARVC are asymptomatic and die suddenly on exertion due to life-threatening ventricular arrhythmia. Other usual symptoms are syncope on exertion, or lightheadedness or dizziness on exertion [6].

ARVC/D leads to sudden death with an estimated 5.4 times greater risk during competitive sports than during sedentary activity [6]. There are several reason that may explain the propensity for ARVC/D to precipitate effort-dependent sudden cardiac arrest. Physical exercise increases the RV afterload and induces RV cavity enlargement, which in turn may elicit ventricular arrhythmias by stretching the RV myocardium and/or favouring re-entrant arrhythmic mechanisms. Myocyte stretching, such as that occurring during training and sports competition, may provoke myocyte death in the presence of genetically defective desmosomes [7].

Another potential mechanism is the "denervation supersensitivity" of the RV to catecholamines [8]. Sympathetic nerves may be damaged and/or interrupted by the RV fibrofatty replacement which distinctively progresses from the epicardium to the endocardium, resulting in a functional denervation and consequent hypersensitivity to circulating catecholamines.

Finally, in a subgroup of patients with familial ARVC/D a cardiac ryanodine receptor (RYR2) missense mutations causing an abnormal calcium release from the sarcoplasmic reticulum has been identified. Wall mechanical stress, such as that induced by exercise, and increased heart rate are expected to exacerbate the cardiac ryanodine channel dysfunction.

Another consideration raises in our patient regarding the occurrence of a sub-febrile temperature for a few days just before death, which suggests possible incident myocarditis as trigger of sudden death. It is known that the ARVC clinical course may present occasional exacerbations with similar clinical picture, without implying incidence of infectious disease.

However, it is worth remembering that trained athletes, after an occasional infectious disease, are usually prone to resume their training precipitously (this has also been the case for our athlete) and do not consistently respect the appropriate convalescence period.

Recommendations for Sports Participation in Patients with ARVC

Athletes with clinical diagnosis of ARVC should be excluded from most competitive sports, with the possible exception of those of low intensity, proven absence of arrhythmias and no incidence of exercise-related symptoms. This recommendation is independent of age, gender, and phenotypic expression of the disease and does not differ for those athletes without symptoms, or treatment with drugs, or interventions with surgery, catheter ablation, or implantable cardioverter defibrillator [9].

On an individual basis, leisure-time physical activity with low dynamic-static intensity may be allowed, such as bowling, cricket, golf. [10].

Finally, neither management with ICD in patients with high risk, nor the presence of a free-standing automated external defibrillator (AED) at sporting events, should be considered absolute protection against sudden death, or treatment strategy, or a justification for participation in competitive sports in athletes with previously diagnosed ARVD/C [9].

References

1. Thiene G, Nava A, Corrado D, et al. Right ventricular cardiomyopathy and sudden death in young people. New Engl J Med 1988, 318:129–133
2. Ahmad F. The molecular genetics of arrhythmogenic right ventricular dysplasia-cardiomyopathy. Clin Invest Med 2003, 26:167–178
3. Corrado D, Thiene G. Arrhythmogenic right ventricular cardiomyopathy/dysplasia: clinical impact of molecular genetic studies. Circulation 2006, 113:1634–1637
4. Brignole M, Alboni P, Benditt DG, Bergfeldt L, Blanc JJ, Bloch Thomsen PE, van Dijk JG, Fitzpatrick A, Hohnloser S, Janousek J, Kapoor W, Kenny RA, Kulakowski P, Masotti G,

Moya A, Raviele A, Sutton R, Theodorakis G, Ungar A, Wieling W. Task Force on Syncope, European Society of Cardiology. Guidelines on management (diagnosis and treatment) of syncope—update 2004. Europace 2004, 6:467–537

5. McKenna WJ, Thiene G, Nava A, Fontaliran F, Blomstrom-Lundqvist C, Fontaine G, Camerini F. Diagnosis of arrhythmogenic right ventricular dysplasia/cardiomyopathy. Br Heart J 1994, 71:215–218

6. Corrado D, Basso C, Thiene G, et al. Spectrum of clinicopathologic manifestations of arrhythmogenic right ventricular cardiomyopathy/dysplasia: a multicenter study. J Am Coll Cardiol 1997, 30:1512–1520

7. Basso C, Czarnowska E, Barbera MD, et al. Ultrastructural evidence of intercalated disc remodelling in arrhythmogenic right ventricular cardiomyopathy: an electron microscopy investigation on endomyocardial biopsies. Eur Heart J 2006, 27:1847–1854

8. Wichter T, Hindricks G, Lerch H, et al. Regional myocardial sympathetic dysinnervation in arrhythmogenic right ventricular cardiomyopathy. Circulation 1994, 89:667–683

9. Pelliccia A, Fagard R, Bjornstad HH, Anastassakis A, Arbustini E, Assanelli D, Biffi A, Borjesson M, Carre F, Corrado D, Delise P, Dorwarth U, Hirth A, Heidbuchel H, Hoffmann E, Melwig KP, Panhuyzen-Goedkoop NM, Pisani A, Solberg EE, Vanbuuuren F, Vanhees L. Recommendations for competitive sports participation in athletes with cardiovascular disease. Eur Heart J 2005, 26:1422–1445

10. Pelliccia A, Corrado D, Bjornstad H, Panhuyzen-Goedkoop N, Urhausen A, Carre F, Anastasakis A, Vanhees L, Arbustini E, Priori S. Recommendations for participation in competitive sport and leisure-time physical activity in individuals with cardiomyopathies, myocarditis and pericarditis. Eur J Cardiovasc Prev Rehabil 2006, 13:876–885

11. Pelliccia A, Culasso F., Di Paolo FM, Maron BJ. Physiological left ventricular cavity dilatation in elite athletes. Ann Intern Med 1999, 130:23–31

Chapter 4
A 32-Year-Old Female Soccer Player with Unexplained Syncope

A.W. Treusch, O. Oldenburg, T. Butz, A. Fründ, E. Oepangat, F. van Buuren, and K.-P. Mellwig

Previous Medical History

This is a 32-year-old female soccer player, suffering of syncope of unknown origin. In the summer of 2001 she had a loss of consciousness while running (the heart rate was reported to be 155–160 bpm). According to her teammates, she was not responding for 2–3 min. The environment temperature was reported to be particularly warm, and general measures were done in the field; she also had infusion therapy, but no hospital admission was advised.

After returning home in August 2001, a general check up at the University Sports Medicine clinic was performed. History revealed previous occurrence 8–10 presyncopal episodes since 2000, without loss of consciousness, during which she was not adequately responding and felt weak for about 2–5 min. She did not report palpitations or dyspnoea on exertion. There was no sign for infection, no tick-bite and no change in exercise conditions. She also reported intermittent vision trouble that occurred during exercise.

Physical Examination and Diagnostic Testing

Cardiovascular physical examination was normal. Blood pressure was 113/82 mmHg and the heart rate was 54/min. Subsequently, diagnostic testing were performed, including 12-lead ECG (Fig. 4.1a,b), which showed sinus rhythm 55 bpm. The QT_c interval was normal. The Sokolow index was negative for left ventricular (LV) hypertrophy. Echocardiography, ECG Holter monitoring, treadmill-testing, and blood chemistry were examined at that time, but no abnormalities were found, and no clear diagnosis could be made.

A.W. Treusch (✉)
Department of Cardiology, Leopoldina Hospital, Gustav-Adolf-Str. 8, D – 97422 Schweinfurt, Germany
e-mail: atreush@hdz-nrw.de

A. Pelliccia (ed.), *Sports Cardiology Casebook*,
DOI 10.1007/978-1-84882-042-5_4, © Springer-Verlag London Limited 2009

(a)

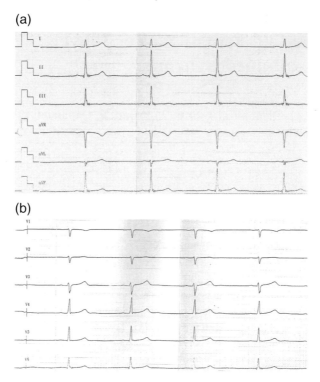

(b)

Fig. 4.1a,b The 12-lead ECG shows sinus rhythm 55 bpm. QT_c interval was normal. QRS-axis between +60 and +90°. Flat T-wave in peripheral lead III with no clinical significance. R/S-change in precordial lead V4. Negative Sokolow index for left ventricular hypertrophy

Clinical Course

In November 2004 during a slow exercise running (while in Turkey for a holiday), she again suffered loss of consciousness. She reported intermittent pre-syncope feeling (like passing-out) with vision difficulties (jittering-view). A possible tongue bite could not be excluded, but no urination and no seizure occurred.

In January 2005 she was admitted at the University Heart-Center for further evaluation. She had not changed lifestyle or exercise conditions. She had suffered from a mild tonsillitis in summer 2004 over 1 week. She reported an intermittent jittering-view which occurred not only during exercise but also on normal walking. An ophthalmologic and neurological examination did not reveal any pathologic condition. Remarkably, the pre-syncope episodes were frequent in 2001 and 2002, but very rare since 2003. Since first presentation at a local sports medicine clinic in 1997, there was no significant change in the clinical presentation of the pre-syncope and syncope.

A previous ECG Holter monitoring recorded in December 1999 showed a few premature ventricular beats (PVBs) during sleeping (199 PVBs, between 10 p.m.

and 3 a.m.) with a heart rate of 45/min. An ECG Holter monitoring in March 2001 showed 66 PVBs and one episode of second degree, type 1 AV-Block at night. No other rhythm disturbances in previous ECG Holter monitoring were seen.

At the time of our evaluation the facts were:

1. Real syncope happened twice in relation to exercise. Both times: first jittering view and colourful view. No flashes or light beams. On second time possible tongue bite.
2. There was no neurological or ophthalmologic cause for the jittering view. We don't know if the jittering view is associated to the syncope.

Family History

She has two sisters, both healthy. Her father is 62 years old and suffers from vocal cord carcinoma and peripheral arterial occlusive disease. He has diabetes type II. Her mother is 52 years old and suffers from myoma of the uterus. There is no family history of myocardial infarction, coronary artery disease, stroke, heart failure or sudden cardiac death.

Type and Level of Sports Activity Performed

Professional soccer player (goalkeeper) in first women's soccer league. Many times German champion and achiever of international awards. Member of German national team and successful participant in World Cup, European Cup and Olympic games. The usual training schedule was 4–5 times per week, twice daily. Competition games are once to twice per week. So far, no relevant injuries associated with sport participation. She takes no medication, no drugs, no contraceptives.

Physical Examination

She was a 32-year-old white female in no apparent distress, alert and oriented to all qualities. Normal body-structure 173 cm, 72 kg, body fat 21%. No relevant findings on head, neck and throat (small tonsils with no signs of infection). Heart was regular in rate and rhythm with 52 bpm. The blood pressure was 110/80 mmHg. Lungs were clear to auscultation. The abdomen showed no relevant findings. No lymph nodes were visible or palpable. A neurological examination showed no abnormalities.

12-Lead ECG

Regular sinus rhythm of 52 bpm. The ECG pattern was normal and unchanged compared to that recorded in 2001 (Fig. 4.2a,b).

Differential diagnostic thoughts and strategies:

(a)

(b)

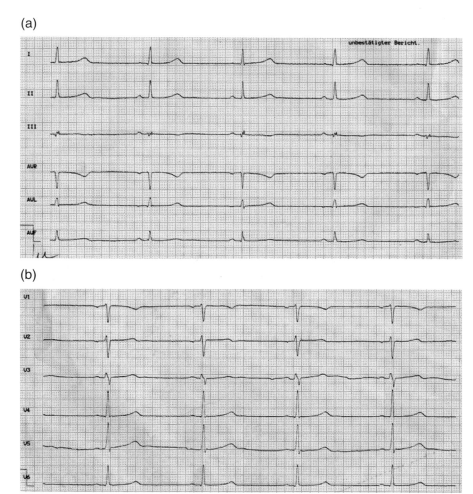

Fig. 4.2a,b The 12-lead ECG recorded in 2005 shows regular sinus rhythm of 52 bpm. The ECG pattern was normal and unchanged compared to that recorded in 2001

- As there was a suspicion for tongue bite, we needed to exclude a seizure or neurological convulsive disease.
- A structural cardiac disease as responsible for syncope on exertion should be excluded, and neuro-cardiogenic syncope should be proved,

Diagnostic Testing

ECG Holter-Monitoring (48 h)

- 40 bpm (at night) – 108 bpm. Average heart rate 59/min. Total: 163 PVBs and 17 PSVBs/24 h, and one couplet of PVBs.

- 42 bpm (at night) – 103 bpm. Average heart rate 52/min. Total: 62 PVBs/24 h. One short run of 3 PVBs. At night a singular episode of second degree, type 1 AV-Block, with pause of 2.5 s, passed asymptomatic.

Blood Pressure (BP)-Monitoring

Day: average systolic BP 116 mmHg (range 103–143)/diastolic BP 74 mmHg (range 63–88)

Night: average systolic BP 112 mmHg (range 105–118)/diastolic BP 66 mmHg (range 61–70)

Late Potentials (HV)-ECG

Bidirectional butterworth filter was set at 40–250 Hz. Total QRS duration was 96.0 ms. Terminal LAS was 33.00 ms and terminal RMS was 55.40 μV for the vector magnitude. There were no late-potentials present (Fig. 4.3).

Exercise – Testing

Test performed on treadmill, starting at 8 km/h. and rising by 2 km/h per 3 min. Exhaustion after 3 min at 14 km/h. Heart rate at rest 81/min, at peak exercise 166/min. Blood pressure at rest 110/87 mmHg, at peak exercise 160/70 mmHg.

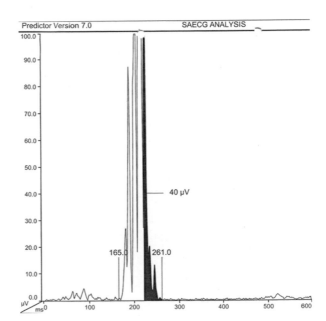

Fig. 4.3 Signal averaging shows the absence of late potentials (HV)-ECG. Bidirectional butterworth filter was set at 40–250 Hz. Total QRS duration was 96.0 ms. Terminal LAS was 33.00 ms and terminal RMS was 55.40 mV for the vector magnitude

Blood pressure and heart rate behaviour was within normal limits. No pathologic ECG changes during exercise were observed.

VO_2 at anaerobic threshold was 41.7 mL/kg/min. Peak VO_2 was 48.7 mL/kg/min, representing 163% of the predicted VO_2-max. Lactate at rest 0.9 mmol/L, at peak 9.3 mmol/L.

In conclusion: no cardio respiratory limitation and excellent physical performance.

Echocardiography

Normal LV cavity dimensions and wall thickness. LV function was normal and no regional wall motion abnormalities were present. No signs of LV hypertrophy. Right ventricle showed normal size and function. No valve abnormalities were found. (Fig. 4.4, Video 4.1).

Ajmalin – Testing

A total of 50 mg Ajmalin (repetitive doses of 10 mg) were infused; there were no ECG changes detectable and, in particular, no ECG sign suggestive for Brugada disease.

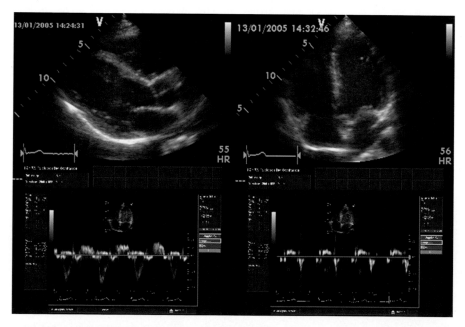

Fig. 4.4 Two-dimensional and Doppler echocardiography shows normal LV cavity dimensions and wall thickness. LV function was normal and no regional wall motion abnormalities were present

Sleep Apnea Monitoring

AHI1/h, RI 2, Apnea index 0/h, Hypopnea index 1/h. No sleep apnea present.

Cardiac CT Scan

There was no evidence for coronary artery anomalies in origin and course, and no sign of atherosclerotic coronary artery disease, namely no stenoses detectable and no relevant calcification (Fig. 4.5).

Cardiac Magnetic Resonance

Normal cardiac dimensions and volumes. Normal LV systolic function, no regional wall motion abnormalities. Mild tricuspid- and aortic regurgitation. The cardiac structures showed no fatty infiltration or other abnormalities. In conclusion, no signs suggestive for ARVD or HCM. (Fig. 4.6, Video 4.2).

Tilt Table Testing

At rest bradycardia with a heart rate of 50/min. Blood pressure 105/60 mmHg. After flipping to 70° upright position, steady rise in heart rate to 85/min in 5 min, the blood pressure did not change until this point while a further rise in heart rate to 115/min was seen. After 12 min (without additional drug provocation), nausea first appeared, then a drop in heart rate (down to 50/min) occurred due to an intermittent AV-Block third degree. At the same time a drop in systolic blood pressure below 50 mmHg occurred. After some seconds, loss of consciousness occurred, followed by a short episode of seizures.

After flipping the patient back to a horizontal position, a fast rise in heart rate and blood pressure were observed. The patient promptly regained consciousness, was awake and oriented to all qualities. No tongue bite. No urination (Figs. 4.7–4.8).

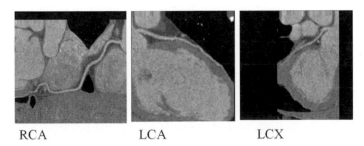

RCA   LCA   LCX

Fig. 4.5 Cardiac CT scan shows normal origin and course of coronary artery, and no evidence of coronary artery disease

Fig. 4.6 Cardiac magnetic resonance shows normal cardiac dimensions and volumes and no evidence of fatty infiltration or other interstitial abnormalities

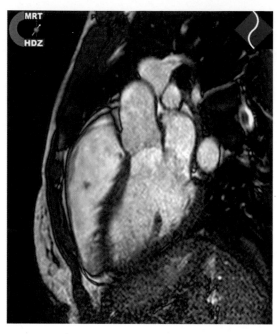

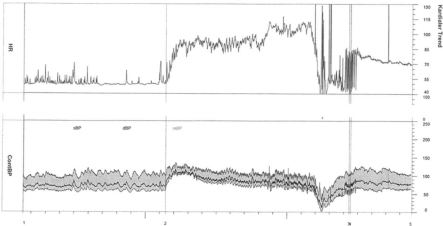

Fig. 4.7 Tilting test. At rest bradycardia with a heart rate of 50/min and blood pressure 105/60 mmHg was recorded. After flipping to 70° upright position, steady rise in heart rate to 85/min in 5 min, the blood pressure did not change until this point while a further rise in heart rate to 115/min was seen

Neurologist Consultation

Neurologist examination was normal and no abnormal findings were found.

On the EEG recording, no extraordinary waves even under photo stimulation and forced hyperventilation were observed. Regular 9.5-Hz alpha activity. Even under

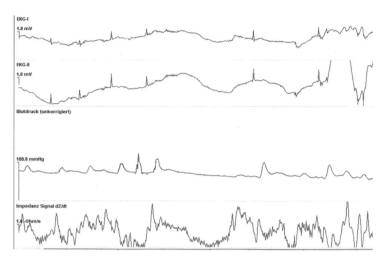

Fig. 4.8 Tilting test (continued). After 12 min (without drug provocation), nausea appeared, then a drop in heart rate (down to 50/min) associated with intermittent AV-Block third degree. At same time a drop in systolic blood pressure below 50 mmHg occurred. After some seconds, loss of consciousness followed by a short episode with seizures occurred

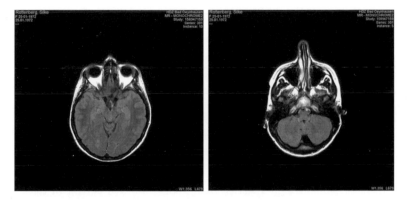

Fig. 4.9 Cerebral MRI shows no evidence for nervous system lesions

sleep-depletion no signs for convulsion or seizure-disease. In conclusion, no pathologic findings were found.

Cerebral Doppler

No stenosis in the carotid and vertebral arteries on both sides were present.

Cerebral MRI

No pathologic findings were present (Fig. 4.9).

Ophthalmologist Examination

Regular view, sight and visus. No pathologic findings.

Laboratory Results

Normal values for electrolytes, liver, renal, CRP, cholesterol, BNP, urinanalysis, WBC, Hb, platelets, coagulation, iron, thyroid and HbA1, HbA1c. Low Ferritin <25 µg/L (normal values 26–120). Negative serologic virus-findings for Coxsackie-, Adeno-, Echovirus. Negative Borreliosis.

Coronary angiography was not done due to excellent quality of the cardiac CT scans. The EP-study was advised but refused by the patient.

Final Diagnosis and Recommendations

In conclusion, the diagnosis was neurocardiogenic syncope without detectable structural cardiac disease. No restriction on sport participation was believed necessary. The patient did not require any medication and only a close follow-up at the local sports medicine clinic was recommended. To date there has been no further syncope episode.

Discussion

Management of athletes with syncope requires careful assessment of the circumstances and sequence of events, in particular the relation with exercise (i.e., during or just after exercise). Therefore, particular care should be spent in collecting the patient's history.

Exercise-induced syncope is relatively infrequent [1–3] and is often associated with an underlying cardiac disease. However, exercise-related syncope may also occur in the absence of underlying cardiac disease, such as was the case here reported, which eventually showed no structural heart abnormality.

This case raised particular concern in view of the implication of our decision on the athlete's career and the need to exclude, with reasonable certainty, the presence of structural cardiac disease as cause of the syncope. Therefore, several diagnostic tests were performed (excessive compared to usual clinical practice) which were consistent in excluding a pathologic heart condition.

The prognosis of neurocardiogenic syncope is reported to be good as long as there is no underlying heart disease [1–3]. Instead, individuals with syncope due to cardiac disease are at increased risk of death from any cause and cardiovascular events in particular.

Previous reports have shown that exercise-induced syncope is not associated with a negative outcome in athletes without cardiovascular diseases or abnormalities [4]. Colivicchi et al. showed that athletes with exercise induced syncope showed a positive response to head-up tilt testing in two thirds of the cases (66.6%). One third had at least one recurrence of exercise-related syncope during follow-up. They came to the conclusion that exercise-related syncope in athletes without cardiac disease is clinically benign, as there was no adverse events in the follow-up [4, 5].

Calkins et al. described the initial symptoms on exercise mediated neurocardiogenic syncope, including nausea, warmth and light-headedness in over 50% of cases. A severe fatigue is also a major initial symptom [6]. If there is a history of syncope in first degree relatives, the likelihood of neuro-cardiogenic origin of the syncope is higher [7]. How to manage the evaluation of syncope is recommended by the European Society of Cardiology task force on syncope [8].

References

1. Soteriades ES, Evans JC, Larson MG, Chen MH, Chen L, Benjamin EJ, Levy D. Incidence and prognosis of syncope. NEJM 2002, 347:878–885
2. Serletis A, Rose S, Sheldon AG, Sheldon RS. Vasovagal syncope in medical students and their first-degree relatives. Eur Heart J 2006, 27:1965–1970
3. Graham LA, Kenny RA. Clinical characteristics of patients with vasovagal reactions presenting as unexplained syncope. Europace 2001, 3:141–146
4. Colivicchi F, Ammirati F, Santini M. Epidemiology and prognostic implications of syncope in young competing athletes. Eur Heart J 2004, 25:1749–1753
5. Colivicchi F, Ammirati F, Biffi A, Verdile L, Pelliccia A, Santini L. Exercise-related syncope in young competitive athletes without evidence of structural heart disease. Clinical presentation and long-term outcome. Eur Heart J 2002, 23:1125–1130
6. Calkins H, Seifert M, Morady F. Clinical presentation and long term followup of athletes with exercise induced vasodepressor syncope. Am Heart J 1995, 129:1159–1164
7. Kosinski D, Bgrubb BP, Karas BJ, Frederick S. Exercise induced neurocardiogenic syncope. Clinical data, pathophysiological aspects, and potential role of tilt table testing. Europace 2000, 2:77–82
8. Brignole M, Alboni P, Benditt D, Bergfeldt L, Blanc JJ, Bloch Thomsen PE, van Dijk JG, et al. Guidelines on management (diagnosis and treatment) of syncope. Task Force on Syncope, European Society of Cardiology. Eur Heart J 2001, 22:1256–1306

Chapter 5
A 23-Year-Old Top-Level Soccer Player Suffering Syncope on Effort

Nicole M. Panhuyzen-Goedkoop and Joep L.R.M. Smeets

Medical History

A 23-year-old male top-level soccer player was referred to our clinic because of recent onset of lightheadedness during training, without loss of postural tone, which lasted for a few seconds. His family history was negative for sudden cardiac death and other known cardiovascular diseases.

Physical Examination

On physical examination blood pressure was normal, 135/75 mmHg, and there were no cardiac murmurs or abnormal heart sounds on auscultation.

12-Lead ECG

The 12-lead resting ECG was within normal limits (Fig. 5.1).

Echocardiography

On transthoracic echocardiography the right and left ventricular morphology was normal, and no evidence of either left or right ventricular dysfunction was observed.

Exercise Electrocardiography

On exercise testing (75 W for 4 min, increment 25 W every 2 min), the athlete reached 350 W with a maximal heart rate of 190 bpm, with a normal rise in blood

N.M. Panhuyzen-Goedkoop (✉)
Department of Sports Cardiology, Sint Maartenskliniek, Location Sports Medical Centre Papendal,
Radboud University Hospital Nijmegen, Arnhem, The Netherlands
e-mail: n.panhuyzen@smcp.nl

A. Pelliccia (ed.), *Sports Cardiology Casebook*,   35
DOI 10.1007/978-1-84882-042-5_5, © Springer-Verlag London Limited 2009

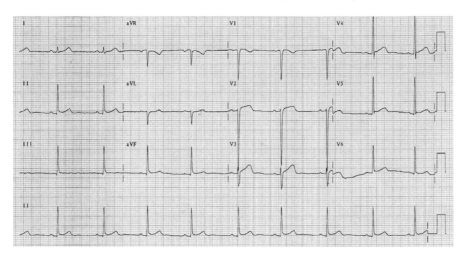

Fig. 5.1 The 12-lead resting ECG shows normal sinus rhythm and normal ECG pattern

pressure. At 330 W, heart rate 175 bpm, a polymorphic couplet of PVBs was seen (Fig. 5.2). During the recovery frequent PVBs mostly with RBBB morphology and superior axis, but also with LBBB morphology and vertical axis, were recorded (Fig. 5.3).

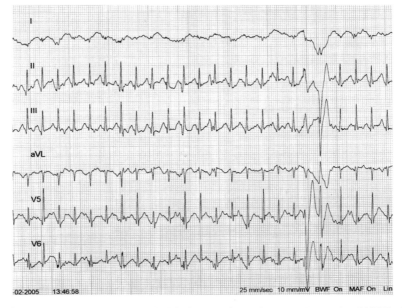

Fig. 5.2 The electrocardiogram recorded during exercise testing, at peak exercise (330 W), showing a couple of polymorphic premature ventricular beats

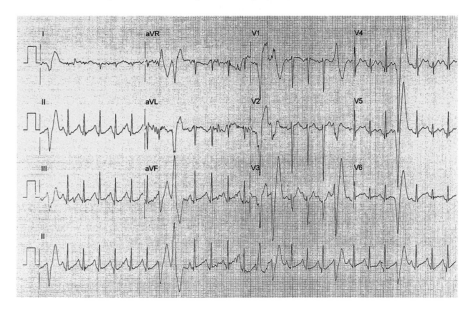

Fig. 5.3 The electrocardiogram recorded during exercise testing, recovery phase, showing isolated premature ventricular beats

Holter Monitoring

Similar PVBs were seen on ambulatory ECG recording during admission. There was no exact information concerning the number of PVBs during 24 h.

Other Diagnostic Testing

In order to exclude with greatest likelihood the presence of structural heart disease, cardiac magnetic resonance (CMR) was performed. CMR demonstrated a normal right and left ventricular morphology and function, and there was no suspicion raised for structural cardiac diseases, such as ARVC, HCM or myocarditis. A signal-averaged ECG was not performed. However, in consideration of the recent onset of the symptoms and with the aim to assess with greater certainty the clinical significance of the presyncopal episode, an electrophysiologic (EP) study was proposed, but rejected by the patient. Given the absence of evident underlying structural cardiac disease, especially ARVC, the patient was allowed to resume training, with the advice to maintain a low intensity schedule.

Clinical Course

Three months later, without premonitory symptoms, he suffered a syncope during a soccer match with brief (8–10 s) loss of consciousness, and spontaneous and complete recovery. At that time, the decision was taken to further investigate the patient in order to assess the arrhythmic risk. The patient gave the informed consent to undergo an EP study.

Other Diagnostic Testing

EP study. Ventricular tachycardia (VT), reproducing the symptoms (dizziness) could easily be induced by stimulation of the right ventricular free wall with three extra stimuli (Fig. 5.4). An attempt to resolve the VT by ablation was performed, but after ablation of the original VT, six other different morphologies of VT originating from RV free wall and apex could easily be induced.

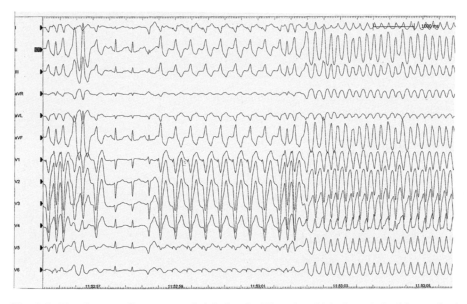

Fig. 5.4 The electrocardiogram recorded during the EP study, which shows inducible sustained VT on stimulation of the right ventricular outflow tract

   Coronary angiography did not reveal significant atherosclerotic lesions and, mostly relevant, excluded the presence of an anomalous origin or course of the coronary arteries.

Treatment

In consideration of the documented right ventricular proclivity for induced VTs, reproducing symptoms, the decision was made to implant an ICD.

Subsequent Clinical Course

Within 3 month of implantation, the athlete again experienced pre-syncope with a documented clinical VT followed by appropriate ICD shock, and prompt resumption of sinus rhythm.

In conclusion, clinical diagnosis in this 23-year-old top-level soccer player with exercise induced pre-syncope (and later syncope), was malignant VT originating from the right ventricular free wall and not associated with detectable structural cardiac disease, especially ARVC, or myocarditis.

Discussion

This young top-level soccer player suffered from exercise-induced syncope. Pre-syncope and syncope on exertion should always be regarded as an alarming sign and must be considered aborted sudden cardiac death until proven otherwise. The incidence of exercise-induced syncope is unknown, but it is predictive of sudden cardiac death within the first year in 16–17% [1, 2].

The history including an exact description of syncope (just before, at onset, during, at end, or after exertion), family history of sudden cardiac death, and measurement of orthostatic blood pressure may give a clue for the diagnosis.

Before diagnosing true cardiogenic syncope, one must exclude cardiac arrhythmias and structural heart disease [3]. In this perspective several investigations may be necessary, including not only echocardiography and exercise testing, but also cardiac magnetic resonance imaging, EP study and coronary angiography [4].

In this young athlete no underlying cardiac cause or familial cause was found during work-up. This illustrates the difficulty in ascertaining the "absence of underlying structural heart disease" which would confer a good prognosis. Exercise testing and Holter monitoring gave a clue for the diagnosis, showing frequent PVBs and exercise-induced couplets, pointing to an arrhythmic problem. During EP study several morphologies could easily be induced in this athlete by stimulation in the right ventricular free wall and outflow tract. PVBs originating from several locations in the right ventricle are common in right ventricular cardiomyopathy. However, there were no imaging criteria for ARVC in this athlete. There was no right ventricular global or regional dilatation on echocardiography or CMR, and there were no typical ECG abnormalities on the 12-lead ECG. Nevertheless, he had inducible sustained VT with a LBBB morphology as the only criterion for the diagnosis of ARVC. Coronary anomaly, channelopathies, HCM and myocarditis were also excluded as an underlying cause. The case shows the importance of thorough cardiovascular evaluation in athletes presenting with exercise-induced symptoms, even if evidence of cardiac morphologic abnormality is lacking and suggests great caution in managing these cases. The same caution should be applied to those cases with syncope and frequent PVCs, because in these instances underlying structural diseases are likely to be found [5]. During ongoing evaluation, athletes should be restricted from continuing competitive sports participation. Even after a negative work-up, a close follow-up and explicit recommendations to the athlete to alert if any premonitory symptoms emerge are mandatory [6].

References

1. Maron BJ, Roberts WC, McAllister HA, Rosing DR, Epstein SE. Sudden death in young athletes. Circulation 1980, 62:218–229
2. Kramer MR, Drori Y, Lev B. Sudden death in young soldiers: high incidence of syncope prior to death. Chest 1988, 93:345–347
3. Brignole M, Alboni P, Benditt DG, Bergfeldt L, Blanc JJ, Bloch Thomsen PE, van Dijk JG, Fitzpatrick A, Hohnloser S, Janousek J, Kapoor W, Kenny RA, Kulakowski P, Masotti G, Moya A, Raviele A, Sutton R, Theodorakis G, Ungar A, Wieling W. Task Force on Syncope, European Society of Cardiology. Guidelines on management (diagnosis and treatment) of syncope—update 2004. Europace 2004, 6:467–537
4. Heidbuchel H, Corrado D, Biffi A, Hofmann E, Panhuyzen-Goedkoop N, Hoogsteen J, Delise P, Hoff PI, Pelliccia A. Recommendations for participation in leisure-time physical activity and competitive sports for patients with arrhythmias and potentially arrhythmogenic conditions. Part II: ventricular arrhythmias, channelopathies and implantable defibrillators. Eur J Cardiovasc Prev Rehab 2006, 13:676–686
5. Biffi A, Pelliccia A, Verdile L, Fernando F, Spataro A, Caselli S, Santini M, Maron BJ. Long-term clinical significance of frequent and complex ventricular arrhythmias in trained athletes. J Am Coll Cardiol 2002, 40:446–452
6. Pelliccia A, Fagard R, Bjornstad HH, Anastassakis A, Arbustini E, Assanelli D, Biffi A, Borjesson M, Carre F, Corrado D, Delise P, Dorwarth U, Hirth A, Heidbuchel H, Hoffmann E, Melwig KP, Panhuyzen-Goedkoop NM, Pisani A, Solberg EE, Vanbuuuren F, Vanhees L. Recommendations for competitive sports participation in athletes with cardiovascular disease. Eur Heart J 2005, 26:1422–1445

Chapter 6
A 21-Year-Old Female Beach Volleyball Player with Palpitations and Pre-syncope on Effort

Nicole M. Panhuyzen-Goedkoop and Joep L.R.M. Smeets

Medical History

A 21-year-old female, top-level beach volleyball player was seen in our clinic because of exercise induced palpitations.

For a few months she had suffered from sudden onset regular rapid palpitations during competition, lasting for a few minutes, followed by lightheadedness and pre-syncope. Before passing out, she managed to ask for a medical time-out. After lying down in a horizontal position for a few minutes the palpitations suddenly ceased and she could resume her match. She reported that during training she felt occasionally the same palpitations, and then stopped her activity for a while, but never had pre-syncope.

A week before presentation to our outpatient clinic she witnessed the sudden cardiac death of a young professional soccer player and she was afraid that she had warning symptoms of dying suddenly. Her family history was negative for sudden cardiac death and arrhythmias.

Physical Examination

The physical examination was normal. The blood pressure in horizontal and standing position was normal (110/65 mmHg).

12-Lead ECG

The 12-lead resting ECG demonstrated a saddle back type like ST-segment elevation in right precordial leads $V_1–V_2$, potentially compatible with type II Brugada syndrome (Fig. 6.1).

N.M. Panhuyzen-Goedkoop (✉)
Department of Sports Cardiology, Sint Maartenskliniek, Location Sports Medical Centre Papendal, Radboud University Hospital Nijmegen, Arnhem, The Netherlands
e-mail: n.panhuyzen@smcp.nl

A. Pelliccia (ed.), *Sports Cardiology Casebook*,
DOI 10.1007/978-1-84882-042-5_6, © Springer-Verlag London Limited 2009

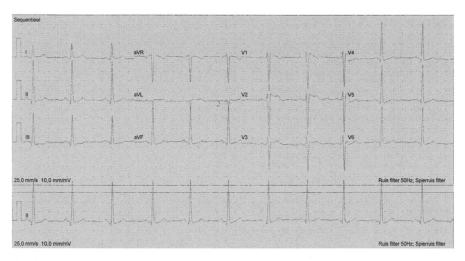

Fig. 6.1 The 12-lead ECG showing ST segment elevation (saddle back type ST elevation) in right precordial leads V₁, V₂ compatible with a Brugada pattern

Diagnostic Testing

She was hospitalized with continuous rhythm monitoring. The next day the 12-lead ECG was normal, and in the right precordial leads there was no more evidence of saddle back type ST-segment elevation (Fig. 6.2).

On echocardiography, right and left ventricular morphology and function were normal, and there was no suspicion for structural heart disease, such as arrhythmogenic right ventricular cardiomyopathy.

During exercise testing (75 W for 4 min, increment 25 W every 2 min), she reached 275 W with a maximal heart rate of 187 bpm (Fig. 6.3). During exercise, a short run of supraventricular tachycardia was seen, compatible with AV nodal reentrant tachycardia (AVNRT), and she recognized the same lightheadedness and pre-syncope as she experienced before.

Carotid sinus massage, Valsalva maneuver and 24-h ECG Holter monitoring did not reveal any supraventricular or ventricular arrhythmia.

The electrophysiologic (EP) study (with three extra stimuli in the right ventricular outflow tract, apex and free wall) was unable to induce ventricular tachycardia. However, during EP study the AVNRT was easily induced with recognizable symptoms of pre-syncope (Fig. 6.4).

Therefore, radiofrequency catheter ablation of the AV nodal slow pathway (part of the reentrant circuit) was performed with success.

Eventually, test with flecainide IV(140 mg) was performed to exclude concomitant presence of Brugada syndrome. The test did not alter the ST-segment pattern in a fashion consistent with Brugada syndrome.

Moreover, SCN5A gene analysis was eventually performed and was negative for mutations compatible with Brugada syndrome.

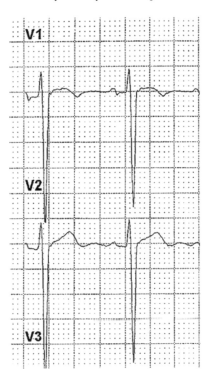

Fig. 6.2 The 12-lead ECG recorded during hospitalization from the same patient as in Fig. 6.1, showing normal ST segment pattern in right precordial leads V_1–V_2

Clinical Course and Recommendations

Three months after the ablation procedure a new cardiac evaluation was performed.

Resting ECG, exercise-ECG and 24-h ECG Holter monitoring could not detect any arrhythmia or any ECG pattern suggestive for Brugada syndrome. Therefore, she was allowed to resume competitive sports.

Subsequent Follow-Up

At 1-year follow-up the cardiac evaluation (including exercise testing and 24-h ECG Holter monitoring) was still negative for inducibility of AVNRT or "Brugada-like" ECG pattern. Meanwhile she was back in international beach volleyball competition without symptoms or any limitations.

In conclusion, this 21-year-old top level female beach volleyball player showed exercise induced AV nodal reentrant tachycardia (AVNRT), correctly identified by ECG and successfully treated with ablation of the slow pathway. The occasional observation of "Brugada-like" ECG pattern in right precordial leads could have been misleading, but reproduction of the symptoms during the induced AVNRT was helpful for definitive diagnosis.

Fig. 6.3a,b The 12-lead ECG recorded during hospitalization from the same patient as in Fig. 6.1. **a** The 12-lead ECG at rest showing normal sinus rhythm. **b** The 12-lead ECG during exertion shows supraventricular tachycardia, compatible with AV nodal reentrant tachycardia (AVNRT)

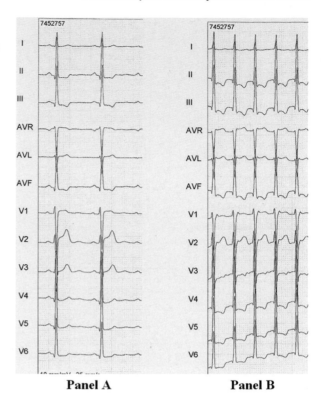

Panel A **Panel B**

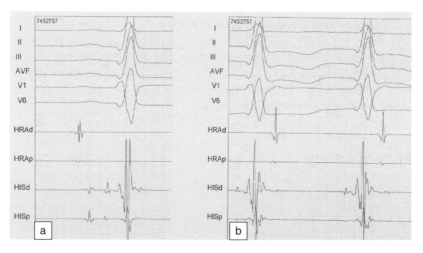

Fig. 6.4a,b The main results of the EP study are shown. **a** Sinus rhythm. **b** Induction of the AVRT. Paper speed 100 mm/s. HRAd = high right atrium distal; HISd = His distal; HRAp = high right atrium proximal; HISp = His prox

Discussion

A detailed patient history is of utmost importance in the diagnostic work-up. This athlete suffered from palpitations during a match and during training. The palpitations were induced by the exercise, thus sympathetic driven. When she continued her physical activity she had lightheadedness and pre-syncope. While in a horizontal position, palpitations ceased abruptly and haemodynamic balance improved. This history was suggestive of paroxysmal tachycardia, which could have been of supraventricular or ventricular origin.

On the 12-lead ECG, a narrow QRS tachycardia, without recognizable P-waves, established the diagnosis of AVNRT. The diagnosis was further confirmed with EP study, which was able to reproduce the symptoms.

AVNRT is the most common reciprocating paroxysmal supraventricular tachycardia, and is often exercise-induced. The recommended therapy in competitive athletes is radiofrequency catheter ablation of the slow pathway. The success rate is over 95%. Catheter ablation outweighs life-long oral medical therapy, which may be prohibited in some sports and/or ineffective [1–3].

This athlete also showed a "Brugada-like" ECG pattern, with incomplete right bundle branch block and a saddle back type ST-elevation in precordial leads V_1 and V_2 (Fig. 6.1). The Brugada syndrome is a sodium channel disorder associated with gene mutation (SCN5A), responsible for syncope and sudden cardiac death due to ventricular tachycardia and fibrillation, usually occurring at night or during vagal stimulation [4]. The ECG pattern typically presents with a ST-segment changes (coved type) in the right precordial leads, while the saddle back type ST-elevation as found in our athlete is not diagnostic for this syndrome. The ECG "Brugada-like" pattern in this case could have been misleading, but other than these non diagnostic ECG changes, there was no evidence of Brugada syndrome in the family, the flecainide test was negative, and research for gene mutation was negative. Our case illustrates how an electrophysiological study may be warranted in many athletes to evaluate the definite arrhythmia mechanism (see also chapter 16).

Summary of the Recommendations for Sports Participation in Athletes with AVNRT [3, 5]

During cardiac evaluation
Restriction of physical activity

1. Ablation

Cardiac evaluation	history, 12-lead -ECG, echocardiography and EP study
Criteria for eligibility	if there is no recurrence of AVNRT >1–3 month, and if there is no underlying cardiac disease
Recommendations	all competitive sports

2. No ablation

Cardiac evaluation	no recurrences >1–3 month, and no underlying cardiac disease
Criteria for eligibility	if AVNRT is sporadic and not exercise-related, and haemodynamics are normal, and no underlying cardiac disease
Recommendations	no sports with increased risk if syncope may occur (such as mountain climbing, motor racing)

References

1. Jackman WM, Beckman KJ, MacClelland HJ, Wang X, Friday KJ, Roman CA, et al. Treatment of supraventricular tachycardia due to atrioventricular nodal reentry by radiofrequency catheter ablation of slow pathway conduction. N Engl J Med 1992, 327:313–318
2. ACC/AHA/ESC Guidelines for the management of patients with supraventricular arrhythmias. Executive Summary. Eur Heart J 2003, 24:1857–1897
3. Heidbuchel H, Panhuyzen-Goedkoop NM, Corrado D, Hoffmann E, Biffi A, Delise P, Blomstrom-Lundqvist C, Vanhees L, Hoffmann PI, Dorwarth U, Pelliccia A. Recommendations for participation in leisure-time physical activity and competitive sports for patients with arrhythmias and potentially arrhythmogenic conditions. Part I: Supraventricular arrhythmias and pacemakers. Eur J Cardiovasc Prev Rehab 2006, 13:485–494
4. Brugada J, Brugada R, Brugada P. The syndrome of right bundle branch block ST segment elevation in V1 to V3 and sudden death – the Brugada syndrome. Europace 1999, 1:155–166
5. Pelliccia A, Fagard R, Bjornstad HH, Anastassakis A, Arbustini E, Assanelli D, Biffi A, Borjesson M, Carre F, Corrado D, Delise P, Dorwarth U, Hirth A, Heidbuchel H, Hoffmann E, Melwig KP, Panhuyzen-Goedkoop NM, Pisani A, Solberg EE, Vanbuuuren F, Vanhees L. Recommendations for competitive sports participation in athletes with cardiovascular disease. Eur Heart J 2005;26:1422–1445

Chapter 7
A 49-Year-Old Male Marathon Runner with Exercise Induced Prolonged Palpitations

Nicole M. Panhuyzen-Goedkoop and Joep L.R.M. Smeets

Family and Personal History

This is a 49-year-old male marathon runner with family history positive for coronary artery disease in both parents, and atrial fibrillation in the father.

Medical History

In the last 12 months the patient experienced unpredictable, intermittent, irregular palpitations during exertion, which lasted for less than 48 h. There were days without any complaints. However, if he had palpitations, it started during running after just few kilometres. The palpitations were accompanied by fatigue and he was not able to continue running or performing maximal exertion.

12-Lead ECG

After 6 months of complaints he consulted a cardiologist elsewhere and a 12-lead ECG was recorded, which revealed sinus rhythm with normal AV conduction, normal QRS complexes and normal repolarization pattern (Fig. 7.1). After 6 months he had the opportunity to reach the outpatient clinic while feeling the complaints above described. On the 12-lead ECG, atrial fibrillation, with average heart rate of 70–80 bpm, was seen (Fig. 7.2). At that time an echocardiography, exercise electrocardiography and blood test were also obtained.

N.M. Panhuyzen-Goedkoop (✉)
Department of Sports Cardiology, Sint Maartenskliniek, Location Sports Medical Centre Papendal, Radboud University Hospital Nijmegen, Arnhem, The Netherlands
e-mail: n.panhuyzen@smcp.nl

A. Pelliccia (ed.), *Sports Cardiology Casebook*,
DOI 10.1007/978-1-84882-042-5_7, © Springer-Verlag London Limited 2009

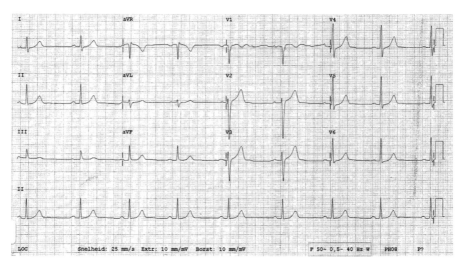

Fig. 7.1 The 12-lead ECG recorded in the absence of symptoms, showed normal sinus rhythm and normal ECG pattern

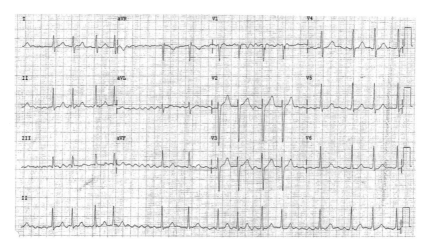

Fig. 7.2 The 12-lead ECG recorded during palpitation showed atrial fibrillation and normal repolarization pattern

Echocardiography

On echocardiography, left ventricular (LV) dimensions were normal (end-diastolic diameter 55 mm, end-systolic 37 mm), but enlarged left atrium was seen (end-systolic transverse diameter 45 mm). LV systolic function was normal (ejection fraction 57%) in the absence of wall motion abnormalities.

Exercise Electrocardiography

The exercise ECG, with standard Bruce protocol, was within normal limits: peak exercise 280 W, maximum heart rate 160 bpm, maximum blood pressure 250/75 mmHg. During the test, sinus rhythm was present, without arrhythmias or conduction abnormalities, and no evidence of ST-T wave changes suggestive for ischemic coronary disease.

ECG Holter Monitoring

The 24-h ECG Holter monitoring revealed sinus rhythm with four short runs (<2 min) of asymptomatic paroxysmal atrial fibrillation at night (Fig. 7.3).

Diagnosis and Treatment

The diagnosis was paroxysmal lone atrial fibrillation. Metoprolol 50 mg a day and oral anticoagulation were prescribed. In addition, treatment with simvastatin 40 mg daily was initiated due to hypercholesterolemia (and xanthelasma).

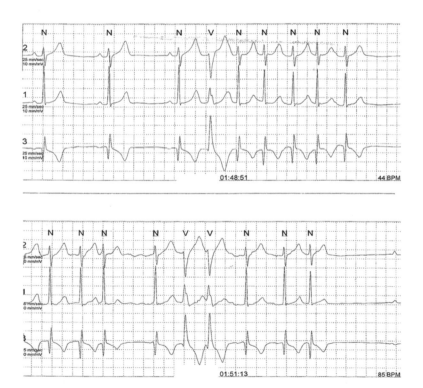

Fig. 7.3 The 24-h ECG monitoring. During the night, short runs of paroxysmal atrial fibrillation were recorded

While on metoprolol he continued his training. However, complaints were progressive, and he could not run for a few kilometres continuously anymore. For this reason, he was referred to our hospital for a second opinion.

2nd Cardiovascular Evaluation

Physical Examination

At presentation the physical examination was normal. Blood pressure was 125/85 mmHg and pulse was regular, with a rate of 100 bpm.

12-Lead ECG

The 12-lead ECG demonstrated atrial flutter (Fig. 7.4).

Other Testing

Echocardiography and myocardial scintigraphy with exercise testing demonstrated diffuse hypo-kinesis with a slightly reduced LV systolic function (ejection fraction 45%). There were no (ir)reversible perfusion defects of the left ventricle.

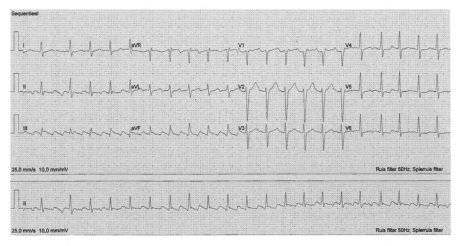

Fig. 7.4 The 12-lead ECG recorded at entry in hospital, showing atrial flutter, with 2:1 conduction and ventricular rate of 142 bpm

Treatment

It was concluded that this 49-year-old athlete suffered from paroxysmal lone atrial fibrillation and a mildly depressed LV function while on ß-blocker therapy given for "rate control". The ß-blocker was withdrawn and he was treated with lisinopril 20 mg daily and sotalol 80 mg b.i.d.

Clinical Course

After 3 months of treatment, the exercise testing was repeated on the treadmill, protocol 6 min 6 km/h, increment 2 km/h every 1 min, until exhaustion. He ran a maximum speed of 17 km/h, with a maximal heart rate (on sinus rhythm) of 165 bpm. His VO2 max was 3.5 L/min (46.6 mL/kg·min), with an equilibrium (R = Q) at 14 km/h, corresponding to a heart rate of 151 bpm. He was allowed to resume training for long distance running and was given the advice to limit his heart rate up to 140 bpm.

For a short period he was able to perform his training three times a week by running an average distance of 10 km, maintaining the heart rate below the advised threshold. Three months later he returned to the out-patient clinic with recurrent complaint, which had started only 1 week before. The patient revealed that he was not able to continue his training adequately and again experienced palpitations on exertion and at rest. At direct inquiry, he revealed that a few weeks before he had ceased taking sotalol. The 12-lead ECG at that time showed atrial flutter.

In consideration that AF deteriorated in persistent AF over time, and there were signs of depressed LV function, a cavo-tricuspid ablation was recommended to prevent fast one-to-one conduction and to control the most symptomatic episodes of atrial arrhythmia. Therefore, the cavo-tricuspid isthmus ablation, after informed consent of the patient, was successfully performed.

After ablation, the 12-lead ECG revealed sinus rhythm with intra-atrial conduction disturbances and a 1st degree AV-block of 220 ms (Fig. 7.5). The patient was discharged from the hospital with treatment including flecainide 100 mg, sotalol 80 mg b.i.d., lisinopril 20 mg, and oral anticoagulation.

Two month after ablation he complained of recurrent symptoms either at rest and on exertion, which lasted less than 1 min. The electrocardiogram recorded during complaints, however, demonstrated sinus bradycardia without evidence of atrial fibrillation or flutter. The 24-h Holter monitoring also showed sinus rhythm (heart rate ranging from minimum of 40 to maximum of 133, mean 63 bpm), without premature supraventricular beats, and with only two premature ventricular beats.

A new complete cardiac evaluation was planned 1 month later (while still in treatment with sotalol 80 mg b.i.d., flecainide 100 mg, lisinopril 20 mg and anticoagulation). On exercise testing he was in sinus rhythm and was able to reach peak exercise of 250 W with maximum heart rate of 154 bpm, with blood pressure 180/80 mmHg. There was no increase in QRS duration during exercise (no "rate dependency"

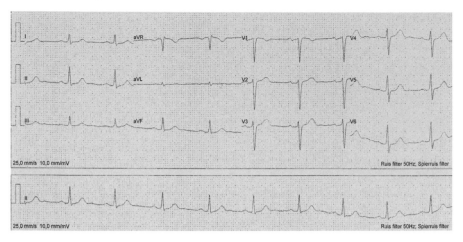

Fig. 7.5 The 12-lead ECG recorded after cavo-tricuspid isthmus ablation showed normal sinus rhythm and 1st degree AV block. Normal repolarization pattern

flecainide). Echocardiography and 24-h ECG Holter monitoring were normal. The decision was taken to withdraw Sotalol and lisinopril. He was advised to resume his long distance running without limitations, under supervision of a sports physician. In the following months the patient did not report further complaints, but his distance training was reduced to no more than 10 km.

In conclusion, this 49-year-old male marathon runner complained of symptomatic paroxysmal atrial fibrillation (PAF). While continuing his training, PAF progressed to persistent atrial fibrillation and atrial flutter (AFl), with a mildly depressed LV function. Treatment with Metoprolol for rate control was not successful, and Sotalol was successful only for a short period. Therefore, the cavotricuspid isthmus ablation was indicated and resulted in the resumption of normal sinus rhythm. However, reduced functional performance was associated with betablocker treatment and persisted after restoration of the sinus rhythm.

Discussion

Exercise induced atrial fibrillation (AF) is reported with apparently larger proportions in adult and senior endurance athletes than in non-athletic populations. The prevalence of AF in the normal population is 0.4–1.0%, and increases with age [1, 2].

Increased sympathetic tone at exertion and increased vagal activity at rest may act as triggers for AF. In individuals prone to develop AF, volume overload is supposed to cause atrial stretching, inducing abnormal atrial refractoriness and facilitating multiple re-entry wavelets which could explain the relation between AF and exercise [1].

When an athlete presents with AF, underlying cardiac causes (such as WPW, cardiomyopathy, myocarditis, coronary artery disease or mitral valve regurgitation) and non-cardiac causes (mainly systemic hypertension) should be investigated and appropriately treated. If no underlying causes are identified, the sport participation under drug treatment may be considered [1, 3].

Rhythm or rate control in young patients with mild or no underlying cardiac abnormality is at present controversial [4, 5]. On a practical basis, rhythm or rate control of paroxysmal AF in athletes is advised according to symptoms and recurrence of AF.

If paroxysmal AF occurs only a few times per year, the athlete could opt for a pill-in-the-pocket approach. Some athletes can prevent sympathetically driven AF episodes by reducing the intensity of exercise below the threshold of inducing AF (heart rate control watch). In symptomatic paroxysmal AF with a reduced exercise tolerance and haemodynamic impairment (syncope, dizziness, fatigue on exertion) negative chronotropic agents are mandatory to prevent symptoms.

When there are frequent recurrences, rhythm control is indicated, as was in this case. However, almost all anti-arrhythmic drugs have a negative effect on exercise performance. ß-Blocker therapy leads to a significant decrease in heart rate and blood pressure and is one of the prohibited substances for some sports on the WADA doping list [6]. On the other hand, it may be essential (at a low dose) to control fast A-V conduction of AF during exercise, which can often not be attained with calcium-channel antagonists or digitalis. When flecainide is necessary this drug should be tested during exercise-ECG for "rate dependent" prolonging of QRS duration, which could be a pro-arrhythmia risk factor and exercise- related sudden cardiac death [7].

Concerning anti-thrombotic management in atrial fibrillation, the current recommendations should be followed [2].

Suggested Recommendations for Sports Participation in Adult and Senior Athletes with Atrial Fibrillation (AF)

During cardiac evaluation
Physical activity should be restricted

1. *First onset of PAF or very sporadic paroxysms*
   If in stable sinus rhythm for > 2 month after paroxysmal AF:

Treatment	"pill in the pocket" approach
Recommendations	all competitive sports allowed
Follow-up	at least yearly

2. *Persistent/permanent AF without major cardiac cause*

Cardiac evaluation:	history, 12-lead resting- and exercise- ECG, echocardiography, Holter monitoring (additional testing according to the case)

Criteria for eligibility: in absence of cardiac disease and WPW, when proven
                               rate control with absence of haemodynamic impair-
                               ment (individualized therapy)
Recommendation   competitive sports allowed on individual basis
Follow-up   at least every 6 month

3. *Atrial flutter*

Cardiac evaluation: history, 12-lead resting- ECG, echocardiography and
                               electrophysiologic assessment.
Treatment: ablation is mandatory
Criteria for eligibility: if asymptomatic for 1 year, competitive sports allowed
                               on individual basis. Resumption of leisure time activity
                               may be anticipated.
Follow-up   at least every 12 month

4. *Paroxysmal AF with secondary cause*

Criteria for eligibility: if secondary to reversible cause, after removal of the
                               cause and there is stable sinus rhythm for > 3 month
Recommendation   eligible for all competitive sports
Follow-up   at least yearly

5. *Oral anticoagulation*

Recommendation   not in athletes engaged in sport with bodily contact or high
                    risk for trauma

References

1. Heidbuchel H, Panhuyzen-Goedkoop NM, Corrado D, Hoffmann E, Biffi A, Delise P, Blomstrom-Lundqvist C, Vanhees L, Hoffmann PI, Dorwarth U, Pelliccia A. Recommendations for participation in leisure-time physical activity and competitive sports for patients with arrhythmias and potentially arrhythmogenic conditions. Part I: Supraventricular arrhythmias and pacemakers. Eur J Cardiovasc Prev Rehab 2006, 13:485–494
2. ACC/AHA/ESC Guidelines for the management of patients with atrial fibrillation. Executive summary Eur Heart J 2006, 27:1979–2030. Full text Europace 2006, doi:10.1093/europace/eul097
3. Pelliccia A, Fagard R, Bjornstad HH, Anastassakis A, Arbustini E, Assanelli D, Biffi A, Borjesson M, Carre F, Corrado D, Delise P, Dorwarth U, Hirth A, Heidbuchel H, Hoffmann E, Melwig KP, Panhuyzen-Goedkoop NM, Pisani A, Solberg EE, Vanbuuuren F, Vanhees L. Recommendations for competitive sports participation in athletes with cardiovascular disease. Eur Heart J 2005, 26:1422–1445
4. Van Gelder IC, Hagens VE, Bosker HA, Kingma JH, Kamp O, et al. A comparison of rate control and rhythm control in patients with recurrent persistent atrial fibrillation. N Eng J Med 2002, 347(23):1834–1840
5. Wyse DL, Waldo AL, DiMarco DP, Domanski MJ, Rosenberg Y, et al. A comparison of rate control and rhythm control in patients with atrial fibrillation. New Eng J Med 2002, 347(23):1825–1833

6. Deligiannis A, Bjornstad H, Carre F, Heidbuchel H, Kouidi E, Panhuyzen-Goedkoop NM, Pigozzi F, Schanzer W, Vanhees L. ESC study group of sportscardiology position paper on adverse cardiovascular effects of doping in athletes. Eur J Cardiovasc Prev Rehab 2006, 13:687–694
7. Crijns HJGM. Changes of intracardiac conduction induced by antiarrhythmic drugs. Thesis 1993. Drukkerij Knoop Haren bv. Haren. The Netherlands

Chapter 8
A Female Cyclist with Prolonged Palpitations on Effort

Pietro Delise, Giuseppe Allocca, Nadir Sitta, Leonardo Coro',
and Massimo Bolognesi

Medical History

This is a 45-year-old, female cyclist with a long term athletic career and very intensive training schedule (average distance: 6,000 km/year). Negative familial history for cardiac disease or events (including premature sudden death) in close relatives. Personal history was unremarkable; in particular, no symptoms or clinical evidence of cardiac disease. For the first time she experienced a prolonged episode of palpitations (lasting for about 1 h) during competition. For this reason, she was referred for cardiac evaluation.

Physical Examination

Physical examination was normal. Blood Pressure was 120/70 mmHg.

Electrocardiogram

The 12-lead ECG showed normal sinus rhythm, without arrhythmia. Mild repolarization abnormalities were noted, including negative T wave in anterior precordial lead V1, and biphasic T wave in V2 (Fig. 8.1).

Echocardiography

The study was performed elsewhere and reported as normal.

P. Delise (✉)
Department of Cardiology, Ospedale di Conegliano, Hospital of Santa Maria dei Battuti, Via Flisati 66, 30171 Mestre (Venezia) Conegliano, Italy
e-mail: pietro.delise@libero.it

A. Pelliccia (ed.), *Sports Cardiology Casebook*,
DOI 10.1007/978-1-84882-042-5_8, © Springer-Verlag London Limited 2009

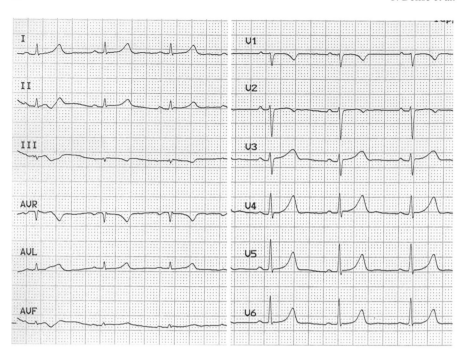

Fig. 8.1 The 12-lead resting ECG showing normal sinus rhythm and normal morphology

ECG Holter Monitoring

A 12-lead Holter monitoring was recorded, and included the usual training session. During effort, the athlete experienced the same palpitations as previously reported. A wide QRS tachycardia with a LBBB pattern and right axis deviation was recorded. The RR interval was 250 ms (corresponding to ventricular rate of 240 bpm) (Fig. 8.2).

Electrophysiological Study

Electrophysiologic (EP) study was then performed. The study (three extra stimuli at two basic cycle lengths of 600 and 400 ms, either at baseline and after administration of 1, 2 and 3 μg/min of Isoprenaline) failed to induce ventricular arrhythmias. The tentative diagnosis was right ventricular outflow tract tachycardia (RVOT).

The eligibility to competitive sport activity was debated between consultant cardiologist and sport medicine specialist. The cardiologist was in favour of continued sport participation, arguing that no heart disease was demonstrable on echocardiography, no ventricular arrhythmia was inducible with EP study, the diagnosis of RVOT conveys a benign prognosis and only sporadic episodes of palpitations had been referred by the athlete. On the other hand, the specialist in sport medicine was

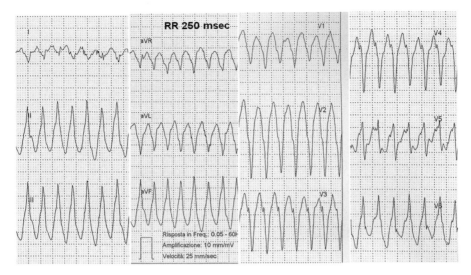

Fig. 8.2 ECG Holter monitoring during the training session, showing a fast (240 bpm) tachycardia with wide QRS complexes. During this episode, the athlete had the same feeling of palpitations, as previously experienced during effort

against competitive sport participation, in consideration that the athlete had recently become symptomatic, that VT induced by effort was recorded and the VT had a short RR interval, concluding that these findings were more consistent with presence of ventricular tachyarrhythmia due to underlying cardiac disease.

Physicians agree to achieve more information regarding the presence of underlying cardiac disease. To the scope, a new echocardiogram with particular attention to right ventricle was requested.

Second Clinical Evaluation

The repeated echocardiogram raised suspicion for mild right ventricular (RV) abnormalities: isolated bulging of RV outflow tract was reported by the observer and the athlete was eventually referred to catheterization.

Coronary angiography showed normal coronary arteries. On right ventriculography, bulging of RV outflow tract and impaired motion of peri-tricuspidal RV wall was observed (Fig. 8.3a,b). Multiple biopsies were taken from different RV segments.

The electro-anatomic voltage map performed with the CARTO showed areas of reduced voltage in correspondence of the RV outflow tract and in the peri-tricuspid wall (Fig. 8.4). The histology showed a pattern of fibro-fatty infiltration which had replaced 60% of RV free wall. Genetic analysis documented a mutation of the gene encoding desmoplakin protein.

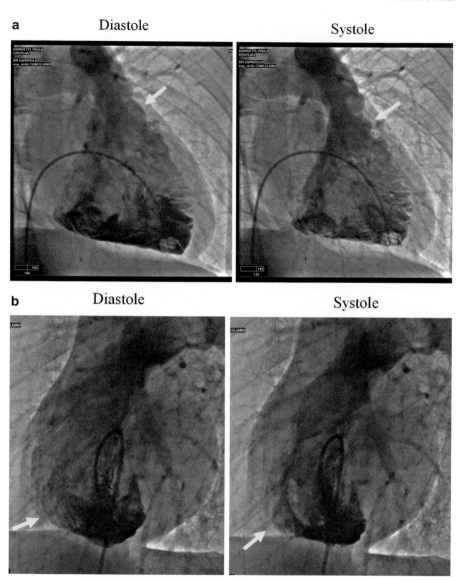

Fig. 8.3a,b **a** Ventricular angiography (*right anterior view*) showed abnormal systolic motion of the right ventricular wall at level of outflow tract (*yellow arrow*). **b** Ventricular angiography (*left anterior view*) showed abnormal systolic motion of the right ventricular wall at level of inflow (peri-tricuspid area) (*yellow arrow*)

Diagnosis and Recommendation

Final diagnosis was arrhythmogenic right ventricular cardiomyopathy (ARVC). The disease was mostly confined to RV outflow tract and peri-tricuspid wall. The athlete was completely informed of the clinical characteristics and outcome of the disease

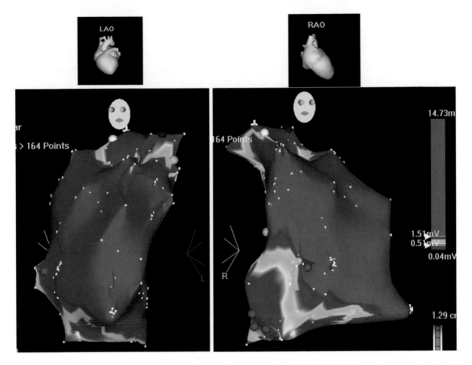

Fig. 8.4 The electro-anatomic map of the *right ventricle* with CARTO showed areas of reduced voltage (*shown in red*) in correspondence of the *right ventricular* outflow tract and peri-tricuspid free wall

and advised to receive an ICD for primary prevention, which she refused. The athlete was then disqualified from competitive sport activity. After 18 months of follow up she is alive and asymptomatic.

Discussion

The diagnosis of ARVC [1–5] was particularly difficult in the present case due to several reasons:

1. There was no familial history of the disease and/or of sudden cardiac death among relatives
2. The 12-lead ECG pattern showed only minor repolarization changes, which could have been misinterpreted
3. There was no evidence of arrhythmia, including premature ventricular beats, preceding the occurrence of VT
4. The athlete had never had symptoms (i.e., syncope) until the first episode of prolonged palpitations which occurred at the age of 45 years

5. The VT was not due to a re-entry, but presumably due to increased automaticity in the outflow tract of the right ventricle, mimicking a benign RVOT

In this case, suspicion of presence of structural cardiac disease was raised mostly by the close relationship of tachyarrhythmia with the effort, as well as by the fast ventricular rate. The electro-anatomic voltage map with CARTO was particularly useful to confirm the segmental RV voltage abnormalities, closely corresponding to abnormal RV segments shown by echocardiography.

This case also raises the issue of the role of continued sport participation in the development (or worsening) of ventricular arrhythmias, which cannot be established with certainty. However, the possibility exists that the chronic hemodynamic overload on the RV associated with high intensive cycling might have promoted the progression of the underlying structural disease and may have triggered the ventricular arrhythmia. For this reason, in accordance with current ESC recommendations, closely resembling in this case the Bethesda Conference #36 [6, 7], it is sound to withdraw these individuals from continued competitive sport activity.

References

1. Marcus FL, Fontane GH, Guiraudon G, et al. Right ventricular dysplasia: a report of 24 adult cases. Circulation 1982, 65:384–398
2. Nava A, Thiene G, Canciani B, et al. Familial occurrence of right ventricular dysplasia : a study involving nine families, J Am Coll Cardiol 1988, 12:1222–1228
3. Corrado D, Thiene G. Arrhythmogenic right ventricular cardiomyopathy/dysplasia: clinical impact of molecular genetic studies. Circulation 2006, 113:1634–1637
4. Nava A, Bauce B. Arrhythmogenic right ventricular cardiomyopathy is a life-threatening disease at high risk for cardiac arrest during effort. Minor forms are as dangerous as major forms? In: Delise P (ed) Controversial and emerging problems in sports cardiology. J Cardiovasc Med 2006, 7:246–249
5. Corrado D, Basso C, Leoni L, et al. Three-dimensional electroanatomical voltage mapping and hystologic evaluation of yocardial substrate in right ventricular outflow tract tachicardia. J Am Coll Cardiol 2008, 51:731–739
6. Pelliccia A, Fagard R, Bjørnstad HH, Anastassakis A, Arbustini E, Assanelli D, Biffi A, Borjesson M, Carrè F, Corrado D, Delise P, Dorwarth U, Hirth A,. Heidbuchel H, Hoffmann E, Mellwig KP, Panhuyzen-Goedkoop N, Pisani A, Solberg E, van-Buuren F, Vanhees L. Recommendations for competitive sports participation in athletes with cardiovascular disease. A Consensus document from the Study Group of Sports Cardiology of the Working Group of Cardiac Rehabilitation and Exercise Physiology, and the Working Group of Myocardial and Pericardial diseases of the European Society of Cardiology. Eur Heart J 2005, 26:1422–1445
7. Maron BJ, Zipes DP. 36th Bethesda Conference: Eligibility recommendations for competitive athletes with cardiovascular abnormalities. J Am Coll Cardiol 2005, 45:2–64

Chapter 9
The Girl with Systolic Murmur on the Left Sternal Border

Mats Börjesson and Mikael Dellborg

Family and Personal History

This 19-year-old female athlete was without history of any clinically relevant disease, except the usual childhood diseases and common colds. The family history was negative for premature cardiac death or congenital heart disease.

She had been training for several years and was competing at national elite junior level in canoeing and was currently enrolled in one of the national sports colleges. For this reason she underwent preparticipation cardiovascular screening according to the recommendations of the European Society of Cardiology [1], which have been implemented in Sweden since 2005 for elite athletes. She filled in a questionnaire and was asked complementary questions by the physician. The athlete was completely asymptomatic.

Physical Examination

The physical examination revealed a normal blood pressure and upon auscultation a previously unreported systolic murmur. The murmur was grade 2/6, audible along the left sternal border with maximum intensity at the third left intercostal space. She was in sinus rhythm and blood pressure was normal. The patient was not on any regular medication.

12-Lead ECG

The 12-lead ECG performed by the examining physician was reported to be normal.

M. Börjesson (✉)
Department of Medicine, Sahlgrenska University Hospital/Östra, Göteborg, Sweden
e-mail: mats.brjesson@telia.com

A. Pelliccia (ed.), *Sports Cardiology Casebook*,
DOI 10.1007/978-1-84882-042-5_9, © Springer-Verlag London Limited 2009

Diagnostic Course

The murmur could be suspected to originate from the right ventricular outflow tract and the pulmonary valve and to be potentially expression of pulmonary valve stenosis, or stenosis of the right ventricular outflow tract or consequence of the increased flow over the pulmonary valve, consistent with intracardiac left-to-right shunts, or extracardiac pathologic conditions such as hyperthyroidism, fever, infection, or pregnancy.

The murmur could also be benign as it may often be heard in young, thin individuals, particularly if they have a low heart rate and a high stroke-volume, such as athletic individuals. To solve the ambiguity of diagnosis, the patient was referred for secondary evaluation to our hospital.

Cardiology Consultation

At cardiology evaluation the physical examination was reported unmodified (as described above). Then the 12-lead ECG and echocardiography were performed.

12-Lead ECG

A standard 12-lead resting electrocardiogram was repeated and was found to be normal (Fig. 9.1).

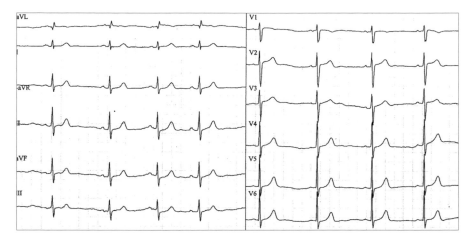

Fig. 9.1 Resting 12-lead electrocardiogram shows normal sinus rhythm. No abnormalities were found

Echocardiography

Trans-thoracic echocardiography (TTE) showed normal left ventricular (LV) morphology and function, normal ejection fraction and no sign of diastolic dysfunction. The ascending aorta, aortic valve and mitral valve were normal, as was the pulmonary and tricuspid valves. The right ventricle showed normal shape and cavity size at the upper limit of normal. From the apical four-chamber view the diastolic diameter of the right ventricle was 34 mm (upper limits in our laboratory: 33 mm). On color-Doppler examination there was a small jet through the atrial septum, from left to right, compatible with atrial septal defect or patent foramen ovale (PFO). Both atria were normal in size.

To confirm the suspicion and characterize the shunt, trans-esophageal echocardiography (TEE) was advised. TEE was preferred to CT-scan, cardiac magnetic resonance, or cardiac catheterization because it requires only light sedation with local anaesthesia and is considered the "gold standard" for detection of atrial septal defects, including PFO.

The TEE described a small PFO, with colour-Doppler signal showing a small, continuous shunt from the left to the right atrium during quiet respiration (Fig. 9.2).

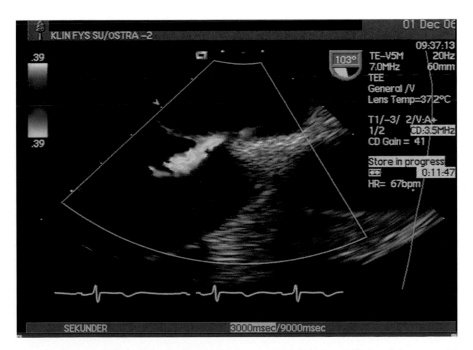

Fig. 9.2 Trans-esophageal echocardiographic view (at 103°) showing the interatrial septum with Color Flow image of small continuous shunt from the *left* atrium (LA) to the *right* atrium (RA) during quiet respiration

Using sonographic contrast (Haemacel), during the Valsalva manouver a right-to-left shunt was evident. The atrial septum was somewhat loose, but did not fulfil the criteria for an atrial septal aneurysm.

Diagnosis

The final diagnosis was a patent foramen ovale, associated with a small left-to-right shunt during resting conditions and with the potential of right-to-left shunting in case of increased right atrial pressure. The murmur may either be a variation of the normal, i.e. a "physiologic" murmur, or related to the somewhat increased flow over the pulmonary valve related to the slight left-to-right shunt.

What is the Risk for Our Patient of Continuing her Sport?

The presence of a PFO in an healthy individual without other pathologic conditions does not indicate any increased risk of embolism and does not require catheter closure. In our athlete, in particular, the PFO carries a very small risk of paradoxical embolization and preventive closure is not indicated, irrespective of participation in high-level athletic activities. Our patient, however, had an unusual feature in that her PFO was constantly open, permitting a small left-to-right shunt. The TTE indicated that the right ventricle was on the upper limit of normal and further follow-up was suggested, with repetition of TTE every 2–3 years. Indeed, high-level athletics may occasionally convey a risk of orthopedic problems and the need for various surgical diagnostic and/or therapeutic procedures. Such procedures may be associated with an increased risk of venous thrombo-embolism and, in that instance, prophylactic treatment to avoid embolism is advisable.

Recommendations

There was no reason to discourage participation in high-level training and competition in our patient [2]. The recommendation was, however, to avoid scuba-diving. In the case of an arthroscopic examination/treatment being necessary, meticulous prophylactic treatment for thrombo-embolism should be given. We also scheduled to repeat TTE, at 2- to 3-year intervals to ensure the atrial shunt does not become significant with volume overload of the right ventricle.

Discussion

The foramen ovale is a canal that shunts oxygenated blood from the right atrium to the left atrium, bypassing the lungs, in the fetus. After birth the changing conditions with pressure being higher in the left atrium than the right close the foramen and in about 75–80% of general population the canal obliterate, without the possibility of subsequent opening. However, in 20–25% of healthy individuals a persistent patent foramen ovale can be found.

The vast majority of people with a PFO does not report symptoms and does not incur cardiac events during life and the discovery of the PFO is often accidental. Nevertheless, the presence of PFO has been reported in a substantial proportion of young people with stroke without other cardiac abnormalities (i.e. cryptogenic stroke). The presumed mechanism for stroke is that a venous thrombus embolizing to the right heart will accidentally, through the PFO, cross over to the systemic circulation and occlude a cerebral artery. This mechanism has been suspected also for severe migraine with aura reported in certain patients. Closure of PFO by catheter techniques is a common, safe method, currently widely recommended for treating young patients with recurrent stroke and/or cryptogenic stroke in the presence of PFO or atrial septal aneurysm, and in patients with a distinct history of paradoxical embolization.

In individuals regularly engaged in scuba diving there is an increased risk of decompression illness. Recurrent decompression illness, primarily in occupational divers, is also an accepted indication for closure.

References

1. Corrado D, Pelliccia A, Bjornstad HH, Vanhees L, Biffi A, Borjesson M, Panhuyzen-Goedkoop N, Deligiannis A, Solberg E, Dugmore D, Mellwig KP, Assanelli D, Delise P, van Buuren F, Anastasakis A, Heidbuchel H, Hoffmann E, Fagard R, Priori SG, Basso C, Arbustini E, Blomstrom-Lundqvist C, McKenna WJ, Thiene G. Cardiovascular pre-participation screening of young competitive athletes for prevention of sudden death: proposal for a common European protocol. Consensus Statement of the Study Group of Sport Cardiology of the Working Group of Cardiac Rehabilitation and Exercise Physiology and the Working Group of Myocardial and Pericardial Diseases of the European Society of Cardiology. Eur Heart J. 2005, 26: 516–524
2. Pelliccia A, Fagard R, Bjørnstad HH, Anastassakis A, Arbustini E, Assanelli D, Biffi A, Borjesson M, Carrè F, Corrado D, Delise P, Dorwarth U, Hirth A, Heidbuchel H, Hoffmann E, Mellwig KP, Panhuyzen-Goedkoop N, Pisani A, Solberg E, van-Buuren F, Vanhees L. Recommendations for competitive sports participation in athletes with cardiovascular disease. A consensus document from the Study Group of Sports Cardiology of the Working Group of Cardiac Rehabilitation and Exercise Physiology, and the Working Group of Myocardial and Pericardial diseases of the European Society of Cardiology. Eur. Heart J. 2005, 26:1422–1445

Chapter 10
Elite Tennis Player with a Complete Atrio-Ventricular Block

Alessandro Biffi, Laura Fiaccarini, and Luisa Verdile

Medical History

This young elite tennis player, 14 years old, was referred for cardiologic evaluation in our Institute (in the year 1977) because of a second-degree atrio-ventricular (AV) block, type 1 observed on resting 12-lead ECG, performed at preparticipation screening. No known cardiovascular disease or symptoms (such as syncope, pre-syncope or dizziness and palpitations) were referred in the medical history. Family history was negative for known cardiovascular disease or sudden death.

Physical Examination

On physical examination he was a healthy male, height 180 cm, weight 78 kg. Blood pressure was 120/80 mmHg. No heart murmurs were detected on auscultation.

12-lead electrocardiogram

Sinus rhythm with heart rate 60 bpm was present. Periods of second-degree AV block, type 1 were observed. Sympathetic-stimulus maneuvers such as hyperventilation, orthostatism and physical exercise caused disappearance of AV block and normalization of the PR interval. In contrast, vagal-stimulus maneuvers, such as Valsalva and eyes compression, showed the worsening of grade of AV block (which transiently become of third degree); see Fig. 10.1.

A. Biffi (✉)
Institute of Sports Medicine and Science, Italian National Olympic Committee, Department of Medicine, Largo Piero Gabrielli, 1 00197, Rome, Italy
e-mail: alessandro.biffi@coni.it

A. Pelliccia (ed.), *Sports Cardiology Casebook*,
DOI 10.1007/978-1-84882-042-5_10, © Springer-Verlag London Limited 2009

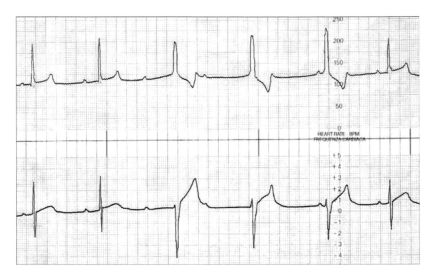

Fig. 10.1 Eyes compression induces the appearance of a third-degree AV block, with periods of AV dissociation and idio-ventricular rhythm

M-mode Echocardiogram

No cardiovascular abnormalities were documented by M-mode echocardiography. Cardiac dimensions were within normal limits and no left ventricular (LV) global dysfunction or wall motion abnormalities were detected.

Electrophysiologic Study

The presence of such advanced AV block in a tennis player was uncommon and unexpected in consideration of the age and level of athletic conditioning. Therefore, to assess the clinical significance of this AV block, i.e., the electrophysiologic mechanisms implicated and the response to provocative stimuli, an electrophysiologic (EP) study was performed. The Hissian electrocardiogram was normal: PA = 20 ms; AH = 120 ms; HV = 40 ms. Incremental atrial pacing (900- to 350-ms cycles) documented a normal recovery time of sinus node; the Wenkebach point was 100 b/m; a dual nodal pathway was identified. Infusion of atropine normalized again the AV node function (Fig. 10.2).

Diagnosis and Recommendation

The diagnosis was transient complete AV block, vagally mediated, in a young trained athlete, without familial or clinical evidence of cardiac disease. Therefore

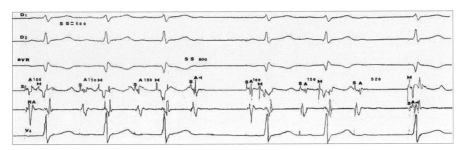

Fig. 10.2 Electrophysiologic study shows the induction of second-degree type 1 AV block during atrial pacing caused by a pre-Hissian delay (prolonged AH interval) with a normal HV interval

the athlete was considered eligible for tennis, with the recommendations to undergo periodical cardiovascular evaluation.

Clinical Course

During the period 1978–1982 the athlete was periodically evaluated in our Institute. Resting ECG showed advanced grade of second degree AV block, type 1, with AV conduction 6:5, 5:4. Again, sympathetic (exercise testing) and vagal maneuvers confirmed the previous response. Pharmacological tests with isoproterenol and atropine induced normalization of AV conduction 1:1, with normal PR interval.

24-Hour ECG Monitoring

A subsequent 24-h ECG Holter monitoring (in 1983) showed a great variability of AV conduction, with periods of first-degree AV block during the day, and nocturnal periods of AV dissociation, associated with wide QRS complexes (Fig. 10.3).

Exercise Testing

In the same year, the athlete was able to perform a maximal exercise test attaining at peak workload 300 W (4 W/kg), with maximal heart rate 172 bpm and blood pressure of 220/85 mmHg, without symptoms or ECG abnormalities. The AV conduction remained within normal limits during the test.

In 1987, at the age of 24 years, he showed no significant changes of AV block with respect to previous findings, and a transient third-degree AV block during night-time with normalization during exercise. Echocardiogram confirmed the absence of structural cardiovascular abnormalities. The athlete had remained completely asymptomatic during the whole period while continuing to be engaged in competitive tennis at elite level.

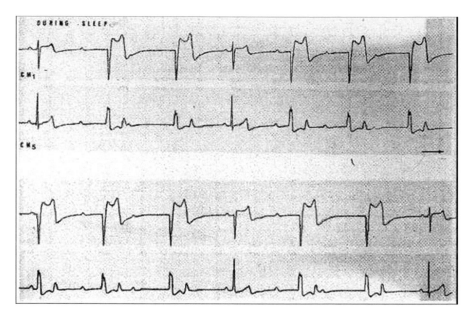

Fig. 10.3 24-h Holter ECG monitoring shows nocturnal periods of third-degree AV block, with wide QRS complexes, and AV dissociation

Clinical Outcome

In 2007 we decided to recall this athlete for a new evaluation after 30 years follow-up. The former athlete was 44 years old and had not taken part in any athletic activity for 15 years.

Medical History

The former athlete referred no cardiovascular symptoms or incidence of cardiovascular abnormalities (either at ECG or echocardiogram) in the last 15 years.

12-Lead ECG

Sinus rhythm 62 bpm, PR interval 0.18 s, normal QRS morphology, absence of arrhythmias and T wave abnormalities (Fig. 10.4).

24-Hour Holter ECG Monitoring

Absence of AV block (even during night-time). Absence of prolonged sinus pauses or any arrhythmias (Fig. 10.5).

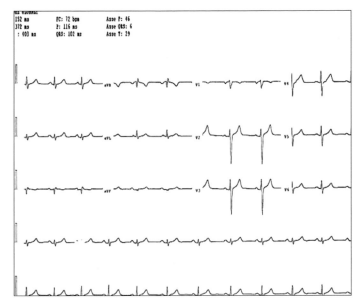

Fig. 10.4 12-lead ECG of the same athlete, at the age of 44 years, after 30 years of follow-up. The ECG is normal, without AV conduction disturbances. The athlete had stopped his competitive sports activity for 15 years and had remained completely asymptomatic during the follow-up period

Doppler-Echocardiography

No structural cardiovascular abnormalities or LV systolic or diastolic dysfunction were detectable.

Discussion

Brady-arrhythmias are common findings in athletic population. They are usually considered a normal variant of athlete's ECG. Sinus bradycardia (<60 bpm) can be found in up to 85% of trained athletes compared to 25% of sedentary subjects [1, 2].

Atrio-ventricular (AV) blocks are also not uncommon in trained athletes: they can be found in up to 35% (first-degree) and 10% (second-degree, type 1) of trained athletes. Mobitz 2 and third-degree AV blocks are occasionally reported in endurance athletes, but are much rarer than second-degree, type 1 (with Wenckebach periods) at 24-h Holter ECG monitoring [3–5]. Brady-arrhythmias are believed to be related to the intensity and length of training in athletes, and reverse when training is reduced or discontinued.

Increased vagal tone is thought to be the basis for most of these arrhythmias. The vagal impact is particularly intense and effective on sinus node and AV node, but

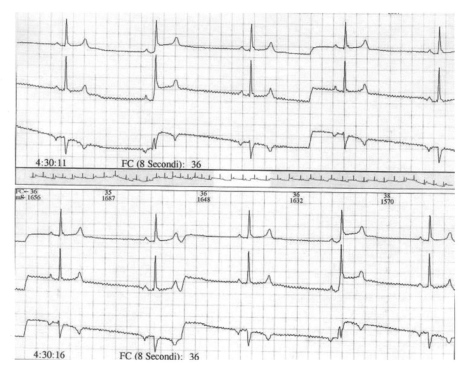

Fig. 10.5 24-hour Holter ECG monitoring after 30 years of follow-up. ECG recording does not show any period of AV block, even during night-time. Only nocturnal sinus bradycardia is documented (36 bpm)

reduction in intrinsic heart rate may be also combined with hypervagotonia. In some cases, however, a genetic predisposition plays an important role in such neurogenic changes [6].

However, AV blocks may also be an expression of structural heart disease, and this option should be carefully considered before assuming AV block to be simply expression of the "athlete's heart syndrome" [7]. This was also our case: we believed that the age of young athlete, the type of sport (tennis and not an endurance sport) and intensity of athletic conditioning were not consistent with the type and degree of AV block found. This consideration moved us to proceed with the diagnostic testing (including EP study), which eventually confirmed the functional origin of the AV block.

Clinical criteria that may be useful in distinguishing between a functional and structural (pathologic) origin of the AV block are: 1. absence of symptoms, such as dizziness or syncope, during a prolonged period of follow-up; 2. disappearance of AV block with exercise, sympathetic drugs or maneuvers; 3. reduction or disappearance of brady-arrhythmias with deconditioning.

In some cases, however, an electrophysiological study may be needed in order to exclude definitely pathologic causes of the AV block, particularly when legal implication regarding eligibility to professional sport activity are under discussion.

References

1. Bjornstadt H, Storstein L, Meen HD, Hals O. Ambulatory electrocardiographic findings in top athletes, athletic students and control subjects. Cardiology 1994, 84:42–50
2. Ferst JA, Chaitman BR. The electrocardiogram and the athlete. Sports Med 1984, 1:390–403
3. Viitasalo MT, Kala R, Eisalo A. Ambulatory electrocardiographic recording in endurance athletes. Br Heart J 1982, 47:213–220
4. Zehender M, Meinetz T, Reul J, Jest H. Electrocardiographic variants and cardiac arrhythmias in athletes: clinical relevance and prognostic importance. Am Heart J 1990, 119:1378–1391
5. Kala R, Viitasalo MT. Atrio-ventricular block, including Mobitz type II-like pattern, during ambulatory electrocardiographic recording in young athletes age 14 to 16 years. Ann Clin Res 1982, 14:53–56
6. Stein R, Moraes RS, Cavalcanti AV, Ferlin EL, Zimerman LI, Riberiro JP. Atrial automaticity and atrio-ventricular conduction in athletes: contribution of autonomic regulation. Eur J Appl Physiol 2000, 82:155–157
7. Zeppilli P, Fenici R, Sassara M, Pirrami MM, Caselli G. Wenckebach second-degree atrio-ventricular block in top-ranking athletes: an old problem revisited. Am Heart J 1980, 100: 281–294

Chapter 11
A Young Canoeist with an Abnormal Electrocardiogram

Fernando Maria Di Paolo, Filippo M. Quattrini, Cataldo Pisicchio, Roberto Ciardo, and Antonio Pelliccia

Family and Personal History

This is a 24-year-old male, elite canoeist, selected on the basis of best athletic results for inclusion in the Italian National Team. Personal history was negative for symptoms and known cardiovascular (CV) diseases. Family history was negative for CV diseases, and no sudden premature deaths had occurred in close relatives.

Physical Examination

The athlete was in good shape and excellent athletic condition; weight was 80 kg, height 185 cm, with a BSA of 2.04 m^2. On physical examination blood pressure was 110/60 mmHg, and no cardiac murmurs or abnormal heart sounds were present.

12-Lead ECG

The 12-lead ECG showed marked sinus bradycardia (35 bpm) with left axis deviation and normal AV conduction (PQ interval: 0.17 s). Markedly abnormal repolarization pattern was evident, with inverted T wave in standard leads II, III, aVF and precordial leads from V1 to V6. The correct QT interval was within normal limits (QTc: 0.43 s) (Fig. 11.1).

F.M. Di Paolo (✉)
Institute of Sports Medicine and Science, Italian National Olympic Committee, Department of Sports Medicine, Largo Piero Gabrielli, 1 00197, Rome, Italy
e-mail: fernando.dipaolo@guest.coni.it

A. Pelliccia (ed.), *Sports Cardiology Casebook*,
DOI 10.1007/978-1-84882-042-5_11, © Springer-Verlag London Limited 2009

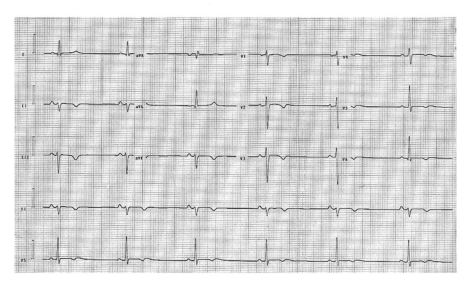

Fig. 11.1 12-lead ECG shows sinus bradicardia (HR 35 bpm), left axis deviation, normal conduction time (PQ interval: 170 ms; QRS: 90 ms; QTc interval: 0.43 ms), diffuse repolarization abnormalities (T wave inverted in precordial leads V1 to V6 and standard leads II, III, and aVF)

Echocardiography

Echocardiographic study showed enlarged LV cavity (end-diastolic diameter = 60 mm), with normal cavity shape and normal systolic function (EF 57%). LV septum and poster free wall were within normal limits (10 mm), there was no segmental LV hypertrophy and no wall motion abnormalities. Left atrium was at upper normal limits (transverse systolic diameter = 40 mm). The diastolic filling pattern, as assessed by transmitral Doppler echocardiography, was normal.

The right ventricle (RV) was mildly enlarged and showed prominent trabeculations, with a mildly enlarged, round-shaped apex. There was no evidence of RV wall motion abnormalities (Fig. 11.2a–d), (Videos 11.1–4). The overall picture did not raise suspicion for either hypertrophic or dilated cardiomyopathy, neither arrhythmogenic right ventricular cardiomyopathy, and was judged consistent with the athlete's heart.

Exercise Electrocardiography

On exercise testing, starting from 50 W for 2 min, with increments of 50 W every 2 min, the athlete reached 300 W at peak exercise, with a maximal heart rate of 155 bpm and blood pressure of 200/80 mmHg. There were no arrhythmia during exertion, no cardiac symptoms, no changes of ST-segment. The abnormal repolarization pattern present in the resting 12-lead ECG improved during exercise, with normalization of the T-wave in precordial leads V2 to V6 (Fig. 11.3).

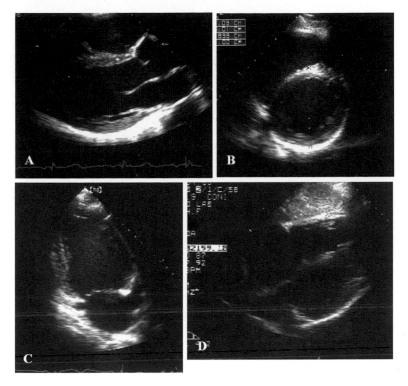

Fig. 11.2a–d Two-dimensional echocardiographic evaluation. **a** Parasternal LV long axis view. **b** Parasternal LV short axis view at papillary level. **c** Two chamber LV apical view. **d** Sub-costal four chamber RV view

ECG Holter Monitoring

The ECG Holter monitoring, including a session of athletic training, showed marked sinus bradycardia at night (minimum HR = 23 bpm), and rare ventricular arrhythmias, characterized by 405 premature ventricular beats (PVBs), one couplet and a short run of ventricular tachycardia (three beats with interval R–R' 290 ms) recorded during physical activity (Fig. 11.4a,b).

Additional Diagnostic Testing

High resolution ECG was performed which showed the presence of late potentials (three criteria: QRS duration: 117 ms; LAS 40: 54 ms, RMS 40: 12 μV); also QT interval dispersion was abnormally prolonged (66 ms) (Fig. 11.5).

In this elite athlete the presence of markedly abnormal ECG pattern, in association with ventricular arrhythmia and the presence of other markers of arrhythmias, such as late potentials, suggested to proceed in the diagnostic course in order to

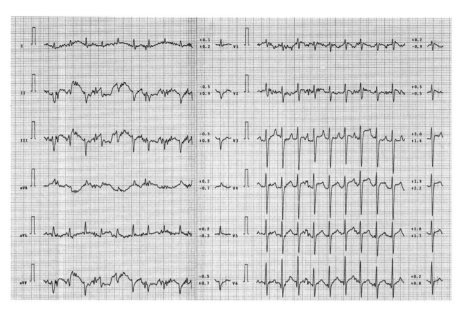

Fig. 11.3 ECG during exercise testing at peak (300 W): heart rate 155 bpm; no alterations of ST-segment and mild improvement of abnormal T wave pattern is evident

evaluate the arrhythmogenic risk and presence of cardiac pathologic condition. During the period the athlete underwent this diagnostic testing, he was withdrawn from training and competitions.

The athlete performed a myocardial scintigraphy that showed normal global and regional perfusion, either at rest and during exercise. The athlete was then referred for electrophysiologic (EP) study. The EP study showed marked sinus bradycardia (minimum heart rate, 29 bpm), the AH time of 100 ms and HV time of 40 ms; a L-W point at 1050 ms with decremental conduction; no retroconduction. These results were interpreted as suggestive for sinus dysfunction of vagal origin, with modest depression of the intrinsic function, and normal nodal conduction time. The programmed ventricular stimulation (double extrastimuli on spontaneous cycle and on driven cycle at 600, 500 and 400 ms, with stimulation on apex and septum) failed to induce ventricular arrhythmias.

Clinical Course

The athlete, during the diagnostic course, despite our advice did not completely stop his training. He felt well, without symptoms, and actually continued with his schedule. One day he went for a canoeing session and never come back. He was found dead at the lakeside.

The autopsy showed increased heart weight (550 g), with normal gross morphology of the LV. The histology of the LV did not show significant lesions. The

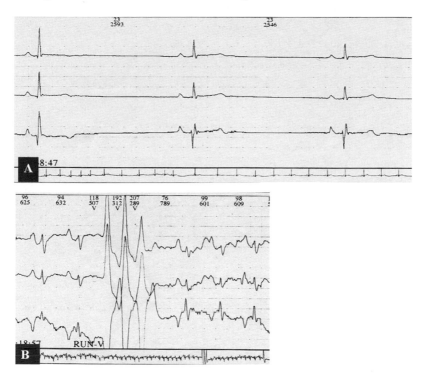

Fig. 11.4a,b ECG Holter monitoring. **a** Nocturnal marked sinus bradycardia (heart rate: 23 bpm).
b Nonsustained ventricular tachycardia (R–R' 290 ms)

RV chamber was dilated, with hypertrophied subendocardial trabeculae, and a diffusely thinned (1.5 mm in thickness) anterolateral wall, in the absence of aneurysm formation. The RV histology showed areas of fibro-fatty replacement of atrophic myocardium. Surviving myocytes were embedded within fibrous tissue and fat (Fig. 11.6). This pattern was consistent with the diagnosis of arrhythmogenic right ventricular cardiomyopathy (ARVC) [1, 2].

Discussion

The death of this elite athlete was a shocking event in consideration of the long-term athletic career, the serial medical evaluations he had undergone during his life, and the high level of achievement he reached during his athletic career. The most compelling question raised by the case was: how was the diagnosis of ARVC missed during life?

Personal and family history were negative and the first and more remarkable finding was the abnormal 12-lead ECG pattern. Several reports over the past 30 years have described a variety of ECG alterations in trained athletes, which have been attributed to cardiac adaptations to systematic athletic conditioning and considered benign expression of the athlete's heart [3]. Therefore the abnormal ECG in this

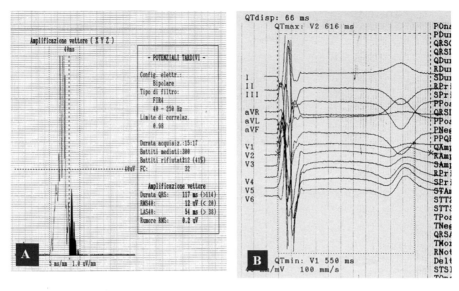

Fig. 11.5a,b **a** Signal averaging ECG: presence of late potentials. **b** QT interval dispersion: positive (QT d: 66 ms)

athlete could have been interpreted as an expression of the athlete's heart. However, the ECG pattern was striking abnormal and the anomalies present here were relatively rare in athletes. In fact, left axis deviation and markedly and diffuse inverted T waves are uncommon findings in athletes (0.1% and 2.7%, respectively) [3]. Therefore, their presence was considered with high suspicion for underlying cardiac disease. However, suspicion for ARVC did not arise specifically because the abnormal T-wave pattern was diffuse in all precordial leads (V1 to V6) rather than confined to anterior leads, as is the case of majority of the young patients with this disease. Athletes with abnormal repolarization patterns in the apparent absence of cardiac disease (such as that observed in this athlete), need serial clinical and imaging testing over a prolonged time period. A substantial minority of these athletes, in fact, may develop phenotypic evidence for arrhythmogenic cardiomyopathies over time with possible adverse cardiac events [4].

Another important finding in this athlete was the ventricular arrhythmia, not frequent, but complex and associated with effort. The arrhythmia was recorded uniquely on Holter ECG monitoring, and we were not able to identify the morphology of PVBs and their origin because a three-leads recording device was used. This experience supports the utility of a 12-leads ECG Holter monitoring in evaluating athletes with ventricular arrhythmia. Other findings suspicious for underlying cardiac disease were the presence of ventricular late potentials, expression of delayed depolarization (late after-depolarization) and prolonged QT interval dispersion, due to delayed conduction between endocardial and epicardial myocardium.

The EP study failed to induce any significant ventricular arrhythmia and was misleading regarding the true arrhythmic risk in this athlete. This experience suggests

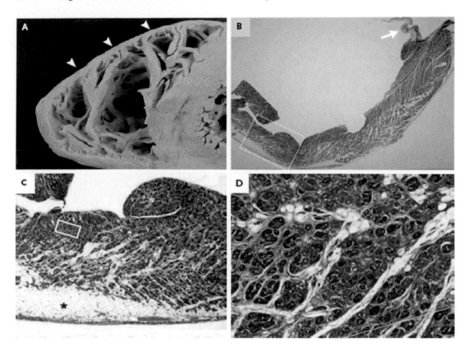

Fig. 11.6a–d Gross and histopathology cardiac findings. **a** Cross section of the heart with a dilated RV chamber, hypertrophied subendocardial trabeculae, and a diffusely thinned (1.5 mm in thickness) antero-lateral wall (*arrowheads*), in the absence of aneurysm formation. **b** Panoramic histologic section of the RV outflow tract, including the pulmonary valve (*arrow*). Abnormalities are not evident in the myocardium (*red staining*) at this magnification (Heidenhain's trichrome stain). **c** Boxed area of **b** at higher magnification, showing areas of fibro-fatty replacement of atrophic myocardium. The *asterisk* indicates epicardial fat, which is regarded as normal. **d** Boxed area of **c** at higher magnification. Surviving myocytes (*red staining*) are embedded within fibrous tissue (*blue staining*) and fat (*white staining*), an acknowledged feature of ARVC

that EP study is not completely reliable to assess the risk for malignant ventricular arrhythmias in young trained athletes, unless a very aggressive (and less specific protocol) is adopted.

The echocardiographic findings (enlarged LV and RV cavity, with normal systolic and diastolic function) were interpreted as expression of physiologic remodeling associated with the athlete's heart [5]. However, while no doubts raised from the analysis of the LV, some doubts might have been raised regarding the right ventricle. An accurate assessment of the RV showed a mildly enlarged cavity, round-shaped apex and prominent cavity trabeculations. These findings would have suggested the utility ofa better morphologic evaluation by cardiac magnetic resonance, which was not available at that time.

Finally, the contemporary presence of electrocardiographic abnormalities and ventricular arrhythmias would had suggested a period of detraining with subsequent re-evaluation [6]. This case illustrates the difficulty of an early diagnosis of ARVC in young asymptomatic individuals. The ARVC diagnosis requires high index of suspicion and specific knowledge of the varied alterations affecting the electrocardiogram and RV morphology. The timely identification of these individuals is a challenge for sports medicine, because ARVC leads to sudden death with an estimated 5.4 times risk in sports compared to sedentary activities [7]. The markedly increased risk associated with sport participation, as well as the lack of consistent and reliable criteria to discriminate the low risk from other patients, are the basis of the current recommendations, which suggest restriction of young individuals with ARVC from competitive sport [8, 9]. This recommendation is independent of age, gender, and phenotypic appearance of the disease and does not differ for athletes without symptoms, or treatment with drugs, or interventions with surgery, catheter ablation, or implantable defibrillator.

References

1. Thiene G, Nava A, Corrado D, et al. Right ventricular cardiomyopathy and sudden death in young people. New Engl J Med 1988, 318:129–133
2. McKenna WJ, Thiene G, Nava A, Fontaliran F, Blomstrom-Lundqvist C, Fontaine G, Camerini F. Diagnosis of arrhythmogenic right ventricular dysplasia/cardiomyopathy. Br Heart J 1994, 71:215–218
3. Pelliccia A, Maron BJ, Culasso F, Di Paolo FM, Spataro A, Biffi A, Caselli G, Piovano P. Clinical significance of abnormal electrocardiographic patterns in trained athletes. Circulation 2000, 102:278–284
4. Pelliccia A, Di Paolo FM, Quattrini FM, Basso C, Culasso F, Popoli G, De Luca R, Spataro A, Biffi A, Thiene G, Maron BJ. Outcomes in athletes with marked repolarization abnormalities on electrocardiogram. N Engl J Med 2008, 358:152–161
5. Pelliccia A, Culasso F, Di Paolo FM, Maron BJ. Physiological left ventricular cavity dilatation in elite athletes. Ann Intern Med 1999, 130:23–31
6. Biffi A, Maron BJ, Verdile L, Fernando F, Spataro A, Marcello G, Ciardo R, Ammirati F, Colivicchi F, Pelliccia A. Impact of physical deconditioning on ventricular tachyarrhythmias in trained athletes. J Am Coll Cardiol 2004, 44:1053–1058
7. Corrado D, Basso C, Rizzoli G, Schiavon M, Thiene G. Does sports activity enhance the risk of sudden death in adolescents and young adults? J Am Coll Cardiol 2003, 42:1959–1963
8. Pelliccia A, Fagard R, Bjornstad HH, Anastassakis A, Arbustini E, Assanelli D, Biffi A, Borjesson M, Carre F, Corrado D, Delise P, Dorwarth U, Hirth A, Heidbuchel H, Hoffmann E, Melwig KP, Panhuyzen-Goedkoop NM, Pisani A, Solberg EE, Vanbuuuren F, Vanhees L. Recommendations for competitive sports participation in athletes with cardiovascular disease. Eur Heart J 2005, 26:1422–1445
9. Maron BJ, Zipes DP. 36th Bethesda Conference: Eligibility recommendations for competitive athletes with cardiovascular abnormalities. J Am Coll Cardiol 2005, 45:2–64

Chapter 12
ECG Repolarization Abnormalities in an African Descent Athlete: Pathologic or Physiologic Finding?

John Rawlins, Peter Mills, and Sanjay Sharma

Medical History

An asymptomatic 17-year-old male African professional soccer player underwent routine medical assessment to screen for pathologic cardiac conditions. The athlete trained for >20 hours (h) and played at least one full competitive soccer game per week. He had no medical or family history of note. Specifically, no premature sudden deaths in close relatives was reported.

Physical Examination

Cardiovascular examination was normal; blood pressure was 110/70 mmHg.

12-Lead ECG

The 12-lead ECG (Fig. 12.1) demonstrated normal sinus rhythm. The R/S wave voltages were increased in precordial leads V3–V6 and met Sokolow-Lyon criteria for LVH, marked (>2 mm) convex S-T segment elevation was evident in precordial leads V1–V4 with T-wave inversion which would warrant further investigation.

Echocardiography

Trans-thoracic echocardiogram demonstrated mild LV hypertrophy with a maximal wall thickness of 13 mm and a non-dilated LV end-diastolic diameter of 50 mm. The left atrial diameter was 38 mm. Indices of diastolic function including Tissue Doppler Imaging velocities were normal (E/A ratio:1.75; E/E' ratio: 6). Systolic function was normal (ejection fraction was 55%) (Fig. 12.2 and 12.3).

S. Sharma (✉)
Department of Cardiology, King's College Hospital, London, Denmark Hill, London, UK. SE5 9RS
e-mail: ssharma21@hotmail.com

A. Pelliccia (ed.), *Sports Cardiology Casebook*,
DOI 10.1007/978-1-84882-042-5_12, © Springer-Verlag London Limited 2009

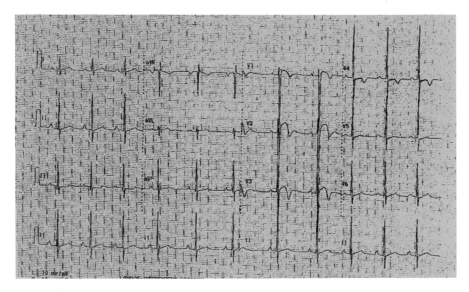

Fig. 12.1 The 12-lead ECGs taken at peak training, showing increased R/S wave precordial lead voltages consistent with LV hypertrophy (Sokolow-Lyon criteria) and marked convex S-T segment elevation in precordial leads V1–V4, followed by T-wave inversion

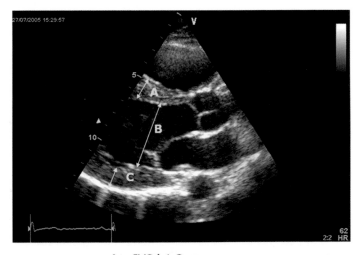

A – IVSd 1.3cm

B – LVEDd 5.0cm

C – PWDd 1.3cm

Fig. 12.2 Echocardiographic parasternal long-axis view from the same athlete, showing a normal LV cavity size, with mild hypertrophy of ventricular septum and posterior free wall

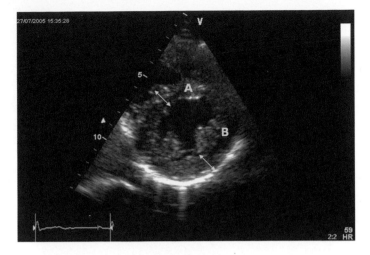

A – IVSd 1.3cm

B – LWTd 1.3cm

Fig. 12.3 Echocardiographic short-axis view from the same athlete, showing an LV cavity size with normal shape and mild symmetric hypertrophy of ventricular septum and free wall. Prominent papillary muscles are also evident

Cardiac Magnetic Resonance (CMR)

CMR with late gadolinium enhancement confirmed mild concentric LVH with a maximal LV wall thickness of 13 mm but did not reveal any features of apical HCM or myocardial fibrosis (Fig. 12.4).

Diagnosis and Recommendations

This athlete exhibited deep T wave inversion on the 12-lead ECG and imaging evidence of LV hypertrophy associated with a non dilated cavity size, which raised suspicion for HCM. The diagnosis of HCM was, however, unlikely due to absence of familial incidence of disease, the intensive training schedule performed, the mild extent of LV hypertrophy associated with normal diastolic function and absence of myocardial fibrosis on cardiac magnetic resonance. In order to resolve the clinical dilemma, he was persuaded to detrain for 8 weeks over the closed season.

Subsequent evaluation demonstrated regression of the marked ECG repolarization abnormalities (Fig. 12.5) and regression of LV mass on cardiac magnetic

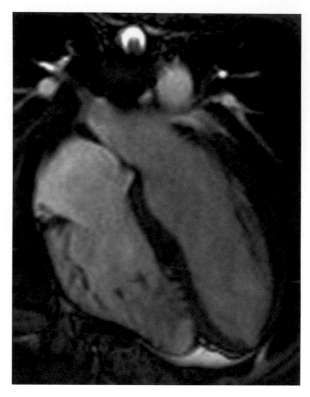

Fig. 12.4 Cardiac Magnetic Resonance imaging. A modified long axis view is shown, demonstrating a structurally normal left ventricle with no evidence of apical hypertrophy

resonance, compatible with diagnosis of physiological LV hypertrophy rather than HCM. The patient was allowed to resume training safely and continue to play soccer at a professional level.

Discussion

Exercise related sudden cardiac death in young (<35) athletes is a rare but well recognised phenomenon. The commonest cause of sudden cardiac death in young athletes in the USA is hypertrophic cardiomyopathy (HCM) [1, 2] and the vast majority of victims are of Afro-Caribbean origin (black) [3]. These events have prompted many sporting organisations in Europe and USA to sponsor independent pre-participation screening programmes to exclude potentially fatal cardiac disorders, prior to acceptance for competition [4]. In parallel, there has been an emergence of a large number of talented black individuals competing at regional and national level in a variety of popular sporting disciplines, notably athletics, soccer

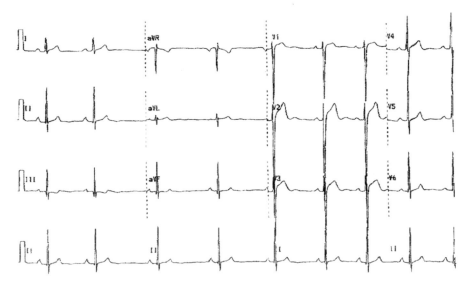

Fig. 12.5 The 12-lead ECG from the same athlete after 8 weeks of complete detraining demonstrating resolution of marked repolarization changes in precordial leads V1–V4

and rugby. For instance, whereas only 2% of the British population is black, 20% of the premier soccer league and up to 25% of the British Olympic squad is black.

The differentiation between physiological LV hypertrophy and HCM is crucial. This differentiation can be challenging in black athletes who may exhibit greater LV hypertrophy when compared to Caucasian athletes participating in identical sporting disciplines. They may also display marked repolarization changes, specifically ST segment changes and deep T wave inversions [5], which may overlap those observed in patients with HCM.

Unfortunately, there are few studies describing criteria for differential diagnosis between physiologic cardiac remodelling and HCM in the black athletic population.

It is uncertain whether ECG and echocardiographic data derived from Caucasian athletes [6] can be extrapolated to black athletes when attempting to differentiate physiological LV hypertrophy from HCM. In the absence of large observational studies in black athletes, there is potential for a false diagnosis of HCM in a black individuals with marked repolarization changes on the ECG and LV hypertrophy on the echocardiogram, resulting in unnecessary disqualification from sport and loss of the many (including economic) benefits derived from sport participation.

There is some evidence that black athletes may exhibit marked repolarization abnormalities, specifically concave ST elevation and deep T wave inversions in the anterior leads that may mimic HCM. One study evaluating 289 collegiate American soccer players, one third of which where black, revealed that 24% of black players demonstrated marked repolarization abnormalities compared with only 8% of Caucasians (p<0.001) [7]. These changes may represent consequence of increased LV mass, reduced sympathetic or increased vagal tone [8, 9]. Recently identified sodium channel polymorphisms amongst the black population [10] may provide a novel explanation for repolarization anomalies observed in these individuals; however, ion channel polymorphisms could not explain the resolution of the electrocardiographic changes with detraining.

There is also evidence that black athletes develop substantially more LV hypertrophy compared to Caucasian athletes. In an echocardiographic study of 280 black American soccer players, 11% of subjects exhibited an LV wall thickness of >13 mm, which could have been consistent with a diagnosis of HCM [11]. Our own experience indicates that 18% of black male athletes exhibit LV hypertrophy (i.e., wall thickness >12 mm) compared with just 4% of sport matched Caucasian athletes of similar age and body size. The racial predilection for developing LV hypertrophy may be due to several mechanisms, such as differences in ACE gene polymorphisms [12], brain natriuretic peptide concentrations, androgen sensitivity and potentially higher exercise-related blood pressure responses in black athletes compared to Caucasian ones.

In conclusion, this case highlights the difficulties in the interpretation of ECG and echocardiographic changes in the Afro-Caribbean/African athlete population. In particular, our athlete exhibited mild LV hypertrophy with non-dilated cavity and associated marked repolarization changes on electrocardiogram which could have been misdiagnosed as HCM. Regression and normalisation of the ECG and LV mass with detraining provided reassurance that these features represented physiological adaptation rather than HCM. This case provides compelling evidence that in some black athletes marked repolarization abnormalities in precordial leads (usually, V1–V3) associated with mild LV hypertrophy are consistent with diagnosis of athlete's heart.

References

1. Maron B, Epstein S, Roberts W. Causes of sudden death in young competitive adults. JACC 1986, 7:204–214
2. Sharma S, Whyte G, McKenna WJ. Sudden death from cardiovascular disease in young athletes; fact or fiction. Br J Sports Med 1997, 31:269–276
3. Maron BJ, Carney KP, Lever HM, et al. Relationship of race to sudden cardiac death in competitive athletes with hypertrophic cardiomyopathy. JACC 2003, 41:974–980
4. Pelliccia A, Fagard R, Bjornstad HH, et al. Recommendations for competitive sports participation in athletes with cardiovascular disease: a consensus document from the Study Group of Sports Cardiology and the Working Group of Cardiac Rehabilitation and Exercise Physiology and the Working Group of Myocardial and pericardial Diseases of the European society of Cardiology. Eur Heart J 2005, 14:1422–1445
5. Walker A, Walker B. The bearing of race, sex, age and nutritional state on the precordial electrocardiograms of young South African Bantu and Caucasian subjects. Am Heart J 1969, 77(4):441–459
6. Maron BJ, Pellicca A, Spirito P. Cardiac disease in young trained athletes. Insights into methods for distinguishing athlete's heart from structural heart disease, with particular emphasis on Hypertrophic cardiomyopathy. Circulation 1995, 91:1596–1601
7. Balady G, Cadigan J, Ryan T. Electrogram of the athlete: an analysis of 289 professional football players. Am J Cardiol 1984, 53:1339–1343

8. Guzzetti S, Mayet J, Shahi M, Mezzetti S, Foale RA, Sever PS, Poulter NR, Porta A, Malliani A, Thom SA. Absence of sympathetic overactivity in Afro-Caribbean hypertensive subjects studied by heart rate variability. J Hum Hypertens 2000 May, 14(5):337–342

9. Serra-Grima R, Estorch M, Carrio I, Subirana M, Berna L, Prat T. Marked ventricular repolarisation abnormalities in highly trained athletes electrocardiograms: clinical and prognostic implications. JACC 2000, 36(4):1310–1316

10. Burke A, Creighton W, Mont E, Li L, Hogan S, Kutys R, Fowler D, Virmani R. Role of SCN5A Y1102 polymorphism in sudden cardiac death in blacks. Circulation 2005, 112: 798–802

11. Lewis JF, Maron BJ, Diggs JA, Spencer JE, Mehrotra PP, Curry CL. Preparticipation echocardiographic screening for cardiovascular disease in a large predominately black population of collegiate athletes. Am J Cardiol 1989, 64:1029–1033

12. Zhu X, Chang YP, Yan D, Welder A, Cooper R, Luke A, Kan D, Chakravarti A. Associations between hypertension and genes in the renin-angiotensin system. Hypertension 2003 May, 41(5):1027–1034

Chapter 13
A 16-Year-Old Female Runner with Prolonged QT Interval

Sandeep Basavarajaiah and Sanjay Sharma

Medical History

A 16-year-old female long-distance runner underwent a cardiovascular evaluation as a part of pre-participation screening programme. She trained approximately 18 h per week and was competing at national level. She was asymptomatic and had no significant past medical history. She denied any regular use of medications or drugs. There was no family history of syncope, premature cardiovascular disease, epilepsy or sudden cardiac death in close relatives.

Physical Examination

There were no stigmata of cardiac disease on physical examination. Her pulse rate was 60 bpm and blood pressure measured on the right upper limb was 120/70 mmHg. Cardiovascular examination was unremarkable.

12-Lead ECG

Her 12-lead ECG showed marked sinus bradycardia of 38 bpm and prolongation of the QT interval (0.62 ms). The corrected QT interval (QTc) was 530 ms, with broad based T-wave morphology (Fig. 13.1).

Other Diagnostic Testing

The patient underwent 48-h Holter monitoring and exercise test to check for other phenotypic features of long QT syndrome, specifically polymorphic ventricular

S. Sharma (✉)
Department of Cardiology, King's College Hospital, Denmark Hill, London, UK SE5 9RS
e-mail: ssharma21@hotmail.com

A. Pelliccia (ed.), *Sports Cardiology Casebook*,
DOI 10.1007/978-1-84882-042-5_13, © Springer-Verlag London Limited 2009

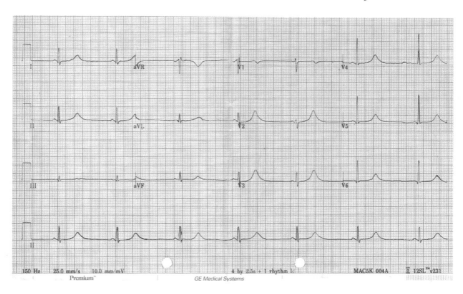

Fig. 13.1 The 12-lead ECG showing a prolonged QTc interval (0.53 ms)

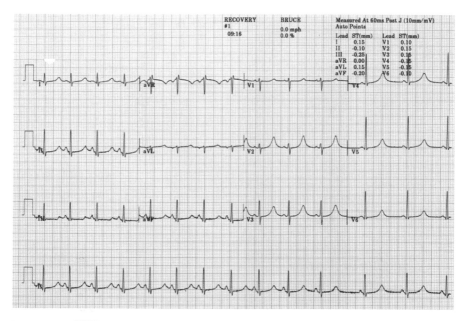

Fig. 13.2 The 12-lead ECG of the same athlete as in Fig. 13.1 demonstrating prolongation of the QTc interval during the recovery phase of exercise

tachycardia (VT) and paradoxical prolongation of the QT interval with increased heart rates. The 48-h ECG Holter recording did not reveal polymorphic VT.

During the exercise testing (performed with the Bruce Protocol), the athlete ran for over 14 min before reaching her predicted maximal heart rate. The QTc interval in the early stages of the exercise test failed to shorten with increasing heart rate and was paradoxically prolonged in the recovery phase at heart rates of 130–100 bpm (Fig. 13.2). She did not develop any arrhythmia (in particular, polymorphic VT) during the test.

Diagnosis and Recommendations

In view of the above findings, she was diagnosed of having long QT syndrome (LQTS). Considering the hereditary nature of the condition, all first-degree relatives (both parents and younger brother) were assessed with a 12-lead ECG.

Her mother had a borderline prolonged QTc interval (460 ms). However, her brother aged 13 years, who was asymptomatic and played regular soccer, also exhibited a markedly prolonged QTc interval of 520 ms on his ECG (Fig. 13.3). Genetic testing was planned to confirm diagnosis, and revealed a mutation in the alpha subunit of the KVLQT1 gene on the chromosome 11, implying the final diagnosis of

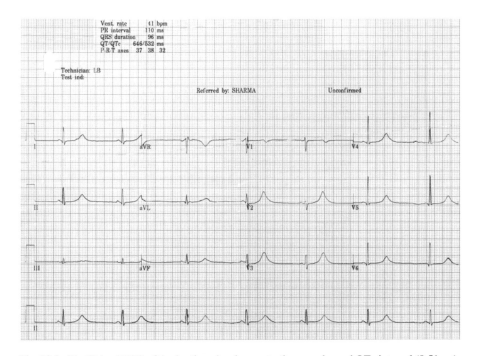

Fig. 13.3 The 12-lead ECG of the brother also demonstrating a prolonged QTc interval (0.51 ms)

congenital LQTS type 1. Both the athlete and her young brother were advised to refrain from all high intensity and competitive sports.

Discussion ensued regarding the indication for ICD; however in view of the absence of symptoms and VT at testing and the negative family history of sudden death, it was decided to treat both individuals pharmacologically with a beta-blocker and follow them up closely, rather than implant an ICD.

Discussion

Congenital long QT syndrome (LQTS) is phenotypic manifestation of a group of inherited cardiac disorders that are caused by mutations within the genes encoding cardiac ion-channels and are characterised by delayed ventricular repolarization, manifested as a prolonged QT interval on the surface ECG above the accepted upper normal limits (0.44 ms in males and 0.46 ms in females). Seven different forms of LQTS are recognised, but LQTS 1-3 account for over 90% of all documented cases [1–3]; LQTS 1 and 2 predispose to exercise mediated polymorphic VT (i.e., torsade de pointes) and are a recognised cause of sudden cardiac death (SCD) in young athletes [1, 2].

Long QT 1 is a result of mutations in the KVLQT1 gene of chromosome 11 that encodes the alpha-subunit of the potassium channel responsible for the slow outward rectifier current (IKs). The role of IKs is to initiate repolarization by opening during the plateau or late phase of action potential. The LQT1 accounts for approximately 40–55% of all congenital LQTS and the arrhythmogenic episodes are mainly triggered by adrenergic surge during physical exertion [4, 5]. Individuals with LQT1 are at highest risk of exercise related sudden death.

The prevalence of congenital LQTS in the general population is estimated to be around 1 in 2,500 to 1 in 10,000 [6, 7]. This figure, however, could underestimate the true prevalence of this syndrome because patients with congenital LQTS can remain asymptomatic or may have only subtle complaints and do not come to medical attention [8]. Indeed, the penetrance of phenotypic features of LQTS on the 12-lead ECG in genetically affected individuals is only 60%. Therefore, 40% of the subjects who harbour the causal genes do not exhibit a prolonged QTc interval on their 12-lead ECG. Finally, individuals with congenital LQTS and other ion-channel disorders have a structurally normal heart and correct diagnosis may be missed at post-mortem examination in several cases of sudden death from LQTS [9, 10].

Pitfalls in the Measurements of QT Interval in Athletes

The QT interval is normally measured from the onset of QRS complex to the point at which the T-wave comes into contact with the iso-electric line. The U-wave is not generally included in the measurement of QT interval. Athletes often exhibit U-waves which may be mistaken for notched T-waves, a recognised manifestation of LQTS. Identification of termination of the T wave in such cases can be particularly difficult. The QT interval should be measured in peripheral or precordial leads, where the terminal pattern of the T wave is clear. However, it is recommended that an apparent U wave exceeding 50% of the T wave probably represents a notched T wave rather than a genuine T-U complex. In such cases the apparent U wave is included in the QTc measurement [11].

Diagnosis of LQTS in Asymptomatic Athletes

Diagnosis based purely upon clinical assessment is clear cut in athletes with a long QTc interval in the context of a family history of the disorder or/and other phenotypic features of this condition, such as polymorphic VT or paradoxical prolongation of the QTc with exercise. In asymptomatic athletes without a family history of LQTS, the diagnosis of LQTS is less straightforward. The Italian pre-participation screening programme comprising of almost 35,000 athletes, recognized 0.7% of athletes based on conventional criteria for a long QTc ($\geq$440 ms in males and $\geq$460 ms in females) [12].

The prevalence of a prolonged QTc interval in highly trained British athletes, based on identical criteria is 0.4% [13]. These figures are considerably higher than those described for hypertrophic cardiomyopathy or arrhythmogenic right ventricular cardiomyopathy. In relation to the relatively high prevalence of a prolonged QTc interval on the 12-lead ECG in athletes, the relatively low death rates from these disorders in athletes suggest either that the vast majority of causal LQTS mutations may be relatively benign, or that most athletes with an isolated long QT interval do not have LQTS.

It is theoretically possible that an isolated long QT interval in an athlete may represent the effect of delayed repolarization due to increased LV mass or the fact that the Bazett's formula may not hold true in individuals with very slow heart rates [14]. In a study of asymptomatic highly trained British athletes a QTc $\geq$500 ms was associated with either paradoxical prolongation of the QT during exercise, an additional phenotypic manifestation of LQT1 and LQT2, or had a first-degree relative with a prolonged QTc interval [13]. Two of the athletes with a QTc $\geq$500 ms scored 4 points on the Schwartz LQT diagnosis scoring system [15] indicating a high probability of LQTS. In contrast, none of the athletes with a QTc >460 ms but <500 ms exhibited any phenotypic features of LQTS and or evidence of familial disease based on the identification of a prolonged QTc in a first degree relative. These observations suggest a QTc >500 ms in an athlete is indicative of unequivocal LQTS and warrants disqualification from most sports to minimise the risk of exercise related SCD. In such cases subsequent genetic testing may be useful in confirming the genotype and facilitating cascade screening if applicable.

The significance of a QTc ranging from 460 to 499 ms in asymptomatic athletes is unknown since genetic testing in this cohort has been limited. Although genetic testing is theoretically possible, the heterogeneity of the disorder allows a genetic diagnosis in about 60% of suspected cases and, indeed, a positive diagnosis may not be available for several months.

Management

Currently, the Bethesda guidelines recommend disqualification from sport in asymptomatic athletic males with a QTc >470 ms and athletic females with a QTc >480 ms [16]. The ESC guidelines are more conservative, warranting disqualification in males with a QTc >440 ms and females with a QTc >460 ms [17].

Gene testing is helpful in management decisions. For example, mutations causing LQT 1 and LQT 2 types represent high-risk in athletes and mandate withdrawal from regular physical training and competitive sport. In contrast, mutations causing LQT3 may be associated with a relatively lower risk for athletic activity, because arrhythmogenic episodes are triggered during bradycardia [5]. In these patients, leisure time physical activity and amateur sport participation can be considered on individual basis.

Athletes who are survivors of sudden cardiac death or those with syncope, documented sustained VT, or a malignant family history of sudden death due to LQTS should receive an ICD [18]. All other athletes are treated with beta-blockers to counteract the potentially fatal effects of adrenergic surges on myocardial early after depolarisations.

References

1. Schwartz PJ, Periti M, Malliani A. The long QT syndrome. Am Heart J 1975, 89:378–390
2. Moss AJ. Prolonged QT syndromes. JAMA 1986, 256:2985–2987
3. Splawski I, Shen J, Timothy KW, et al. Spectrum of mutations in long-QT syndrome genes: KVLQT1, HERG, SCN5A, KCNE1, and KCNE2. Circulation 2000, 102:1178
4. Schwartz PJ. The long QT syndrome. Curr Probl Cardiol 1997, 22:297
5. Schwartz PJ, Priori SG, Spazzolini C, et al. Genotype-phenotype correlation in the long-QT syndrome: gene-specific triggers for life-threatening arrhythmias. Circulation 2001, 103:89
6. Quaglini S, Rognoni C, Spazzolini C, Priori SG, Mannarino S, Schwartz PJ. Cost-effectiveness of neonatal ECG screening for the long QT syndrome. Eur Heart J 2006, 27:1824
7. Vincent GM, Timothy KW, Leppert M, et al. The spectrum of symptoms and QT intervals in carriers of the gene for the long-QT syndrome. N Engl J Med 1992, 327:846
8. Napolitano C, Priori SG, Schwartz PJ, et al. Genetic testing in the long QT syndrome: development and validation of an efficient approach to genotyping in clinical practice. JAMA 2005, 294:2975
9. Basavarajaiah S, Shah A, Sharma S. Sudden cardiac death in young athletes. Heart 2007, 93(3):287–289
10. Schwartz PJ, Stramba-Badiale M, Segantini A, et al. Prolongation of the QT interval and the sudden infant death syndrome. N Engl J Med 1998, 338:1709
11. Al-Khatib SM, LaPointe NM, Kramer JM, Califf RM. What clinicians should know about the QT interval. JAMA 2003, 289:2120

12. Corrado D, Basso C, Schiavon M, Thiene G. Screening for hypertrophic cardiomyopathy in young athletes. N Eng J Med 1998, 339(6):364–369
13. Basavarajaiah S, Wilson M, Whyte G, Shah A, Behr E, Sharma S. Prevalence and significance of an isolated long QT interval in elite athletes. Eur Heart J 2007, 28:2944–2949
14. Moss A. Measurement of the QT interval and the risk associated with QTc prolongation: a review. Am J Cardiol 1993, 72:23B
15. Priori SG, Schwartz PJ, Napolitano C, Bloise R, Ronchetti E, Grillo M, Vicentini A, Spazzolini C, Nastoli J, Bottelli G, Folli R, Cappelletti D. Risk stratification in the long-QT syndrome. N Engl J Med 2003, 348(19):1866–1874
16. Maron BJ, Isner JM, McKenna WJ. Twenty-sixth Bethesda conference: recommendations for determining eligibility for competition in athletes with cardiovascular abnormalities. Task Force 3: hypertrophic cardiomyopathy, myocarditis and other myopericardial diseases and mitral valve prolapse. J Am Coll Cardiol 1994, 24(4):880–885
17. Pelliccia A, Corrado D, Bjornstad HH, Panhuyzen-Goedkoop N, Urhausen A, Carre F, Anastasakis A, Vanhees L, Arbustini E, Priori S. Recommendations for participation in competitive sport and leisure-time physical activity in individuals with cardiomyopathies, myocarditis and pericarditis. Eur J Cardiovasc Prev Rehabil 2006, 13(6):876–885
18. Groh WJ, Silka MJ, Oliver RP, et al. Use of implantable cardioverter-defibrillators in the congenital long QT syndrome. Am J Cardiol 1996, 78:703

Chapter 14
Athlete with Variable QTc Interval and Abnormal T Wave Pattern

Emanuele Guerra, Filippo M. Quattrini, and Antonio Pelliccia

Family and Personal History

This was a 16-year-old female swimmer, selected for inclusion in the national team and referred to the Institute of Sport Medicine and Science for medical and cardiologic evaluation before participation in world championships. Personal history was negative for symptoms or previous cardiovascular disease. Family history was positive for diabetes. No known cardiac disease or sudden cardiac deaths were reported in close relatives.

Physical Examination

Athlete was in good physical and athletic condition; weight was 65 kg, height 180 cm. Blood pressure was 125/75 mmHg. No murmurs or abnormal heart sounds were detectable on cardiac auscultation.

12-Lead ECG

The 12-lead ECG showed sinus bradycardia (mean heart rate 43 bpm) with normal QRS axis, normal AV conduction (PQ:0.14 s). The QT interval duration was 0.46 s, and corrected QT interval (QTc) was 0.39 s. The R/S wave voltages were normal, but negative T waves were evident in precordial leads V_2 to V_6. (Fig. 14.1).

E. Guerra (✉)
Institute of Sports Medicine and Science, Italian National Olympic Committee, Largo Piero Gabrielli, 1 00197 Rome, Italy
e-mail: casaguerra@alice.it

A. Pelliccia (ed.), *Sports Cardiology Casebook*,
DOI 10.1007/978-1-84882-042-5_14, © Springer-Verlag London Limited 2009

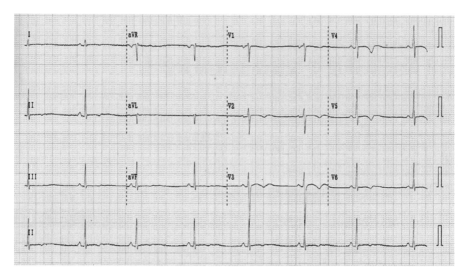

Fig. 14.1 The 12-lead ECG at first evaluation, showing marked sinus bradycardia, and abnormal repolarization pattern with T-wave inversion in precordial leads V_2–V_6

Echocardiography

Left ventricular (LV) cavity size was within normal limits (51 mm), and wall thickness was normal, without evidence of segmental hypertrophy. Prominent trabeculations were observed in the apical region, close to the antero-lateral and postero-inferior wall (Fig. 14.2a,) (Video 14.1). LV systolic function was normal (ejection fraction 60%) without evidence of wall motion abnormalities. Diastolic filling, as assessed by transmitral Doppler flow, was normal. The right ventricular (RV) chamber was within normal limits, and there were no morphologic or segmental RV abnormalities.

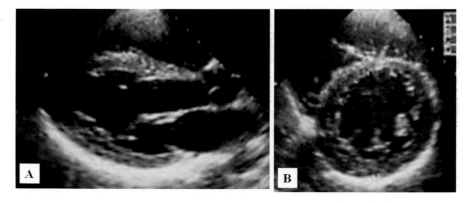

Fig. 14.2a,b **a** Parasternal long-axis view. **b** Parasternal short-axis view.

Video 14.1 Parasternal long axis and short axis views; prominent trabeculations in the antero-lateral and postero-inferior wall are evident, at level of papillari muscle and LV apex

Exercise Electrocardiography

On exercise testing, starting from 30 W for 2 min, with 2-min step and 30-W workload increments, the athlete reached 180 W, with a peak heart rate of 169 bpm and blood pressure of 165/70 mmHg. No arrhythmias and no symptoms were induced by exertion. The abnormal repolarization pattern observed in the resting 12-lead ECG partially resolved during exertion (Fig. 14.3).

ECG Holter Monitoring

ECG Holter monitoring was performed, including a session of athletic training. The ECG showed bradycardia during night (minimum heart rate:34 bpm) and the presence of rare premature supraventricular beats (PSVBs). The abnormal T wave pattern was present for most part of the ECG recording, with partial resolution during physical activity.

This athlete showed abnormal repolarization pattern in the absence of evident cardiac disease. Question raised regarding the clinical significance of the prominent trabeculations present in the LV apex, i.e., a subtle variant of cardiomyopathy,

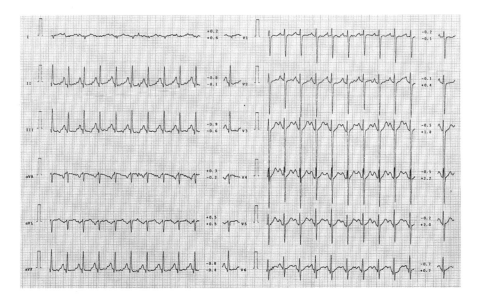

Fig. 14.3 Exercise test. The abnormal repolarization pattern partially resolved during exertion

such as LV non compaction. For this reason, we extended our testing with evaluation of the family members and additional imaging testing (cardiac magnetic resonance).

Family Screening

The mother showed a trabeculation pattern in LV cavity which echoed the morphology seen in the athlete. Otherwise, 12-lead ECG was unremarkable and personal and family history were negative (Fig. 14.4a,b) (Video 14.2).

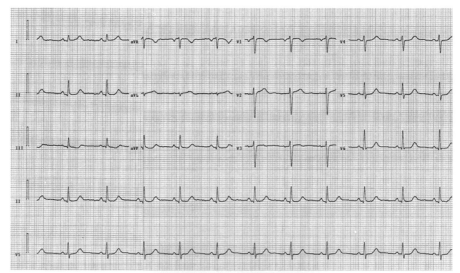

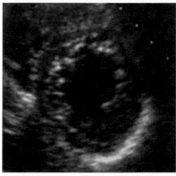

Fig. 14.4a,b   a Athlete's mother 12-lead ECG showed normal pattern. **b** Athlete's mother echocardiography showed trabeculation pattern similar to that observed in the athlete

Video 14.2   Athlete's mother echocardiography showed trabecular pattern within the LV cavity similar to that observed in the athlete

Cardiac Magnetic Resonance

Cardiac magnetic resonance showed either left and right ventricular chambers of normal morphology and dimensions, with LV wall thickness within normal limits. No evidence of focal or diffuse alterations of signal intensity within myocardium was observed at delayed enhancement with post-gadolinium. The examination confirmed the presence of trabeculations in the apical region of both ventricles, without evidence of non-compaction myocardium. No global or segmental LV dysfunction was seen and, finally, the epicardial course of both coronary vessels was regular (Figs. 14.5 and 14.6).

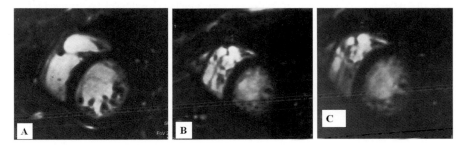

Fig. 14.5a–c Cardiac magnetic resonance. LV chamber imaged at level of papillary muscle (**a**), more distal level (**b**) and LV apex (**c**). Normal cavity dimensions and shape are evident, with trabeculation in mid-distal segments of the LV

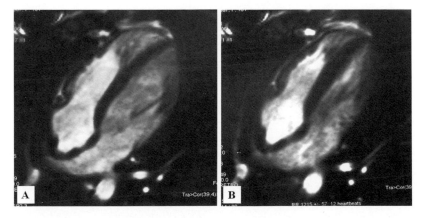

Fig. 14.6a,b Cardiac magnetic resonance. **a** Diastole. **b** Systole. *Left* and *right* ventricular chambers are imaged. Normal LV and RV cavity dimensions and shape are evident, with trabeculation in mid-distal segments of the LV

Diagnosis and Recommendations

In consideration that abnormal ECG pattern in this athlete was not an expression of underlying cardiac disease, based on the imaging testing and negative family screening, that the athlete had no arrhythmia, no symptoms, and showed excellent adaptation to exertion, we cleared her for competitions, with the obligation of a periodic cardiovascular evaluation.

Clinical Course

The athlete continued in her successful competitive career and underwent periodical controls in our Institute. At the age of 19 years, the 12-lead ECG showed marked sinus bradycardia and, for the first time, a prolonged QT interval (absolute QT = 0.52 s, corrected QT interval = 0.47 s). The abnormal repolarization pattern present in previous ECG tracings had remained substantially unchanged.

An ECG Holter monitoring was repeated, which confirmed the presence of transiently prolonged QTc interval, with wide range of values, from 0.39 to 0.55 s (Fig. 14.7). On exercise testing the athlete reached 240 W, with a peak heart rate of 166 bpm and blood pressure 180/75 mmHg. No arrhythmias were induced by

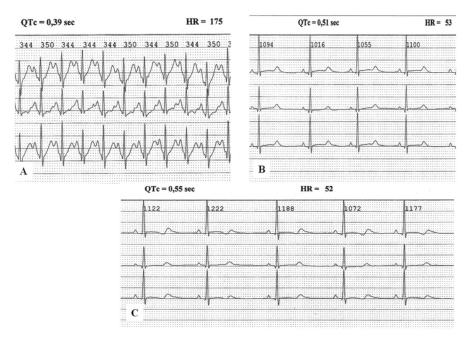

Fig. 14.7a–c ECG Holter monitoring showing wide variability of the QTc interval, with values ranging from 0.39 s (**a**) to 0.51 s (**b**) up to 0.55 (**c**)

exertion, and no symptoms. The abnormal repolarization pattern resolved almost completely during exertion. At that time, question of Long QT syndrome (LQTS) raised, and the athlete was referred to an expert consultant to assess the presence of genetic anomalies responsible for the LQTS.

Genetic Analysis

DNA analysis for gene mutations associated with LQTS was therefore performed. Namely, KCNQ1, KCNH2, SCN5A genes were assessed with denaturing high performance liquid chromatography. The investigation failed to show any abnormalities in these genes potentially responsible for LQTS.

Follow-Up

The athlete has continued her successful career with a commitment to undergo periodical controls. At the most recent evaluation, the athlete was in good physical condition, without symptoms and no events during the overall follow-up. The physical examination was normal, and there were no cardiac murmurs or abnormal heart sounds.

The most recent 12-lead ECG showed marked sinus bradycardia (heart rate:37 bpm) with normal AV conduction (PQ interval:0.14 s). The QTc interval duration was 0.44 s. The R/S wave voltages in precordial leads were normal, and the abnormal repolarization pattern was mildly improved (i.e., inverted T wave only in precordial leads V_2–V_3). On exercise testing, there were no arrhythmia and no symptoms and QTc interval reduced to 0.40 s. The abnormal repolarization pattern showed complete resolution during effort, as shown before. The ECG Holter monitoring showed rare isolated SVPBs and one couplet. Again, the QTc interval showed a wide QT variability, with QTc values ranging from 0.43 to 0.53 s. No changes were seen in the cardiac morphology, as assessed by echocardiography.

Although a reasonable explanation for the large QTc variability and abnormal repolarization pattern was not evident to our evaluation, we nevertheless considered that over a prolonged time period no clinical or diagnostic evidence had emerged for cardiomyopathy in the candidate (and in the family). Therefore, we believe that there were no sufficient reasons to disqualify this athlete from competitions. The athlete is still engaged in sport practice with high level of achievements and undergo periodical cardiovascular controls (every 6 months.)

Discussion

The case described here presents two points of major interest, i.e., the abnormal repolarization pattern and the prolonged QTc interval. With regard to the repolarization abnormalities, this finding is not uncommon in young, trained athletes [1, 2]. The clinical significance of these electrocardiographic changes, in the absence of structural cardiac disease, is debated and incompletely resolved. However, our experience suggests that abnormal repolarization on 12-lead ECG may represent the initial and sole expression of underlying cardiomyopathies, which become evident many years later and that may be cause of adverse outcomes [2]. Therefore, a serial accurate control is needed in these athletes to identify timely those (few) who may incur clinically evident cardiac disease and prevent adverse events.

The athlete described in the present case did undergo serial cardiovascular evaluations, including repeated imaging testing (echocardiography and cardiac magnetic resonance) which failed to show structural cardiac changes supporting diagnosis of HCM (or other cardiomyopathies). The unique morphologic peculiarity observed in this athlete (and in the mother) was the prominent trabecular pattern present in the LV apex. This pattern was not considered to be an expression of non-compaction myocardium, but possibly a variance of the normal LV morphology and deprived of clinical significance, although we cannot exclude that it may be responsible for the abnormal repolarization pattern observed in the athlete's ECG.

The other point of interest was the prolonged QTc interval in this athlete. Repeated measurements of QTc interval showed a wide spectrum of values, occasionally above the accepted normal limits (i.e., 0.44 ms in males and 0.46 ms in females). Congenital long QT syndrome (LQTS) is a phenotypic manifestation of a group of inherited cardiac disorders caused by mutations in the genes encoding potassium cardiac ion-channels, characterized by delayed ventricular repolarization. The prevalence of congenital LQTS in the general population is between 1/2,500 and 1/10,000 [3, 4].

Diagnosis of LQTS is commonly made on the basal electrocardiogram, with QT interval measured from the beginning of QRS complex to the point at which the T-wave intercepts the iso-electric line. U-waves may often be mistaken for notched T-waves, which could be a manifestation of LQTS. It's sometimes hard to recognise termination of the T wave, so the QT interval should be measured where the terminal pattern of the T wave is clear. However, penetrance of phenotypic features of LQTS on the 12-lead ECG in genetically affected individuals may be not complete and, therefore, proportion of genetic positive individuals do not exhibit a prolonged QTc interval on 12-lead ECG.

For this reason, DNA analysis for gene abnormalities associated with LQTS is recommended, in order to confirm diagnosis of LQTS in borderline or controversial cases. However, the heterogeneity of the disorder allows a genetic diagnosis in up to 60% of suspected cases; this implies that a substantial minority of the potentially affected individuals are, at present, not detectable by current genetic analysis [3, 4].

The influence of athletic training and sport participation on the QTc interval is unknown. However, a relatively longer QTc interval is reported in trained athletes and occurrence of QTc interval above the widely used upper limits (0.44 s in males or 0.46 s in females) is not an uncommon finding in young trained athletes [5]. While the prevalence of a prolonged QTc interval on the 12-lead ECG in athletes is relatively high, incidence of sudden death from these disorders in athletes is pretty rare. Such data suggest that the vast majority of causal LQTS mutations may be relatively benign, or more likely that most athletes with an isolated prolonged QTc interval do not have LQTS.

In a study of asymptomatic highly trained British athletes the QTc interval ≥500 ms was associated with either paradoxical prolongation of the QT during exercise (an additional phenotypic manifestation of LQT1 and LQT2), or first-degree relatives with a prolonged QTc interval [5]. The study suggests that a QTc >500 ms in the 12-lead ECG is indicative of unequivocal LQTS and warrants disqualification from most sports to minimise the risk of sudden death.

Gene testing has been considered to be helpful in management decisions. For example, mutations causing LQT 1 and LQT 2 types represent high-risk in athletes and mandate withdrawal from regular physical training and competitive sport. In contrast, mutations causing LQT3 may be associated with a relatively lower risk for athletic activity, because arrhythmogenic episodes are triggered during bradycardia [3, 4]. However, in the clinical practice no such subtle distinctions are usually made and, according the ESC recommendations, unequivocal diagnosis of LQTS conveys the recommendation to withdrawn athlete from competitive sports [6].

References

1. Pelliccia A, Maron BJ, Culasso F, Di Paolo FM, Caselli G, Biffi A, Piovano P. Clinical significance of abnormal electrocardiographic patterns in trained athletes. Circulation 2000, 102: 278–284
2. Pelliccia A, Di Paolo F, Quattrini F, et al. Outcomes in athletes with marked Ecg repolarization abnormalities. N Engl J Med 2008, 358:152–161
3. Vincent GM, Timothy KW, Leppert M, et al. The spectrum of symptoms and QT intervals in carriers of the gene for the long-QT syndrome. N Engl J Med 1992, 327:846
4. Schwartz PJ, Priori SG, Spazzolini C, et al. Genotype-phenotype correlation in the long-QT syndrome: gene-specific triggers for life-threatening arrhythmias. Circulation 2001, 103:89
5. Basavarajaiah S, Sharma S, et al. Prevalence and significance of identifying an isolated long QTc interval in elite athletes. Eur H J 2007 Dec 28(23):2944–2949
6. Pelliccia A, Fagard R, Bjørnstad HH, Anastassakis A, Arbustini E, Assanelli D, Biffi A, Borjesson M, Carrè F, Corrado D, Delise P, Dorwarth U, Hirth A, Heidbuchel H, Hoffmann E, Mellwig KP, Panhuyzen-Goedkoop N, Pisani A, Solberg E, van-Buuren F, Vanhees L. Recommendations for competitive sports participation in athletes with cardiovascular disease. A consensus document from the Study Group of Sports Cardiology of the Working Group of Cardiac Rehabilitation and Exercise Physiology, and the Working Group of Myocardial and Pericardial diseases of the European Society of Cardiology. Eur Heart J 2005, 26:1422–1445

Chapter 15
Young Triathlete with Unusual ST-Segment Elevation in Precordial Leads

Luisa Verdile, Filippo M. Quattrini, Fernando Maria Di Paolo, and Antonio Pelliccia

Family and Personal History

This is a 28-year-old male athlete engaged in triathlon, selected for inclusion in the Italian National team. According to the program of the Italian National Olympic Committee, he was referred to our Institute for a comprehensive medical and physiologic evaluation. The family history was negative for cardiovascular disease and/or sudden death in relatives. Personal history was negative for any previous event or cardiovascular symptom. Athlete also denied drugs abuse.

Physical Examination

The athlete was in good physical shape and athletic condition. Weight was 61 kg and height 171 cm, with a BSA of 1.71 m^2. On physical exam, the blood pressure was 110/70 mmHg and there were no murmurs or abnormal heart sounds.

12-Lead ECG

The 12-lead resting ECG showed sinus bradycardia (47 bpm), left QRS axis deviation, first-degree atrioventricular block (PR interval: 0.23 s). QRS voltages were increased in precordial leads V3 to V5. The QRS duration was 0.09 s, and QT interval correct with Bazzet formula was at upper limits (QTc: 0.45 s).

An rSr' pattern was present in anterior precordial leads V1–V2. Indeed, an unusual ST-segment elevation was present in precordial leads. Specifically, in lead V2, a ST-segment elevation of about 2 mm was present at J point, followed by

L. Verdile (✉)
Institute of Sports Medicine and Science, Department of Cardiology, Largo Piero Grabrielli, 1 00197 Rome, Italy
e-mail: luisa.verdile@coni.it

A. Pelliccia (ed.), *Sports Cardiology Casebook*,
DOI 10.1007/978-1-84882-042-5_15, © Springer-Verlag London Limited 2009

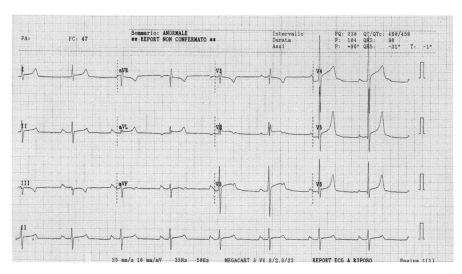

Fig. 15.1 Baseline 12-lead ECG of the athlete showing rSr' pattern in anterior precordial leads V1–V2. In addition, ST-segment elevation was present in precordial leads V2–V6 and standard leads I and aVL. Specifically, in lead V2, the ST-segment elevation was of 2 mm at J point, followed by down-sloping ST-segment and inverted T wave. In precordial lead V3 the ST-segment pattern was convex type, continuing with a positive, notched T wave. In precordial leads V4–V6 the ST-segment showed upward concavity and a positive, tall terminal T-wave

down-sloping ST segment and inverted T wave. In precordial lead V3 the ST-segment pattern was convex, continuing with a positive, but notched T wave (Fig. 15.1).

Exercise Electrocardiography

On exercise testing, starting from 50 W for 2 min, with increment of 50 W every 2 min, athlete reached 450 W, with a maximal heart rate of 166 bpm and a blood pressure of 210/85 mmHg. During exercise the shortening of PR-interval was observed (to 0.16 s). The incomplete right bundle branch block and the down-sloping ST-segment in precordial leads V1, V2 did not show significant changes during exercise. No arrhythmias and no symptoms occurred during exertion (Fig. 15.2).

The particular pattern of ST segment elevation (down-sloping and continuing with inverted/notched T wave) observed in precordial leads raised question of appropriate interpretation, i.e., possible expression of Brugada ECG pattern. Although diagnosis of Brugada syndrome appeared to be less likely than an early repolarization pattern (which is commonly seen in young athlete population), we were forced to exclude presence of Brugada syndrome, because of the implications related to sports eligibility. Therefore, sodium channel blocker testing was planned.

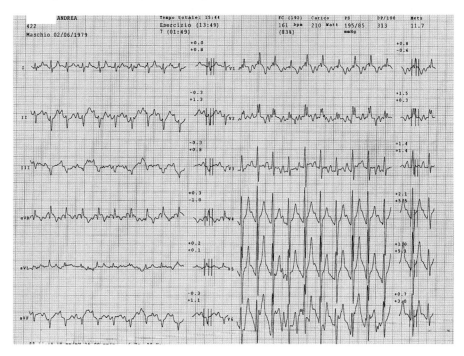

Fig. 15.2 12-lead exercise ECG in the same athlete showed presence of rSr' pattern and ST-segment elevation in precordial leads V1, V2, without significant changes of the down-sloping pattern seen at rest and followed by a clearly inverted T wave

Flecainide Testing

The test was performed with flecainide infusion 0.1 mg/kg in 5 min with continuous ECG monitoring. After drug infusion, the heart rate was 50 bpm, PR interval 230 ms, QRS interval 104 ms, QTc interval 400 ms. The ST segment elevation in precordial leads was <1 mm without significant changes into true "coved type" pattern. The test was considered negative for Brugada syndrome. The ST-segment elevation in this athlete was therefore considered to be an innocent early repolarization and consistent with physiologic remodeling of the athlete's heart.

Echocardiography

Left ventricular (LV) septum and posterior free wall were at upper normal limits (12 and 11 mm respectively), without evidence of segmental hypertrophy. LV cavity dimension was within normal limits (transverse diameter 53 mm), and so global systolic function (EF 60%), without wall motion abnormalities. The diastolic filling pattern, as assessed by trans-mitral Doppler echocardiography and Tissue Doppler Imaging, was normal. The right ventricle showed a normal cavity dimension, with a rich trabecular pattern and no wall motion abnormalities (Video 15.1).

Video 15.1 Long axis, short axis and apical four chamber and subcostal views of the cardiac morphology and function in the same athlete. The overall picture was consistent with a physiologic adaptation to the athlete's training schedule

Diagnosis

In conclusion, this athlete showed an ECG pattern which raised suspicion for Brugada pattern and required provocative testing to clarify diagnosis, specifically to exclude that syndrome. The final diagnosis was early repolarization and, therefore, no restrictions were placed on sport participation.

Discussion

Several studies over the past 30 years have described a variety of ECG alterations in trained athletes (including, most frequently, sinus bradycardia, first-degree atrioventricular block, increased QRS voltages suggestive for LV hypertrophy, early repolarization pattern). These alterations have been judged to be physiologic cardiac adaptations to systematic athletic conditioning [1].

Not unusually, however, ECG alterations in trained athletes may mimic those observed in patients with heart diseases. In particular, the ST-segment elevation in anterior precordial leads may occasionally be suggestive for Brugada Syndrome, such as in this athlete.

Brugada syndrome is a genetic arrhythmogenic cardiac disease, with an autosomal dominant pattern of transmission, characterized electrocardiographically by a typical pattern of ST-segment elevation in the anterior precordial leads, right bundle branch block morphology, and clinically by syncope and/or sudden cardiac death [2, 3].

The genetic alteration causing Brugada syndrome has been demonstrated in mutations in SCN5A, the gene encoding for the cardiac sodium channel, also responsible for the LQT3 subtype of long QT syndrome [3]. The typical ECG pattern of the Brugada syndrome is characterized by a ST-segment elevation in the right precordial leads (usually, V1 to V3), of >2 mm with coved morphology, followed by a negative T wave. This pattern (type 1) is diagnostic for the disease (Fig. 15.3). In a substantial number of patients, this pattern is not present on the baseline ECG, but is inducible by provocative testing with sodium channel blockers. In patients with Brugada syndrome also different repolarization patterns may be found, i.e., ST-segment elevation with saddleback morphology and high take-off ST-segment elevation of >2 mm, followed by either positive or negative terminal T wave (type 2). Finally, a type 3 has also been described, with either a coved or saddleback morphology with ST-segment elevation of <1 mm (Fig. 15.3).

Diagnosis of Brugada syndrome is definitive when the typical type 1 ST-segment elevation is observed in >1 right precordial lead (V1 to V3) in the presence or absence of a sodium channel–blocking agent (such as flecainide or ajmaline), and in

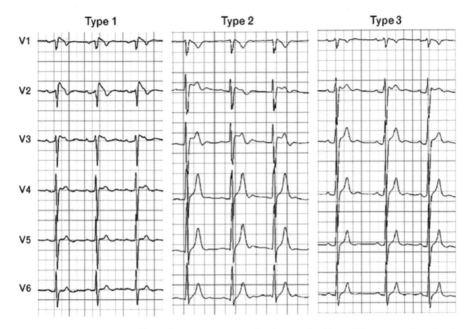

Fig. 15.3 The three ECG Brugada patterns. Type 1 is characterized by a ST-segment elevation in the right precordial leads, of >2 mm with coved morphology, followed by a negative T wave. Type 2 pattern is characterized by ST-segment elevation with saddleback morphology and high take-off ST-segment elevation of >2 mm, followed by either positive or negative terminal T wave. Type 3 pattern shows either a coved or saddleback morphology with ST-segment elevation of <1 mm. Only type 1 is diagnostic for the disease

conjunction with documented ventricular fibrillation (VF), polymorphic ventricular tachycardia (VT), syncope, family history of sudden cardiac death at young-adult age (<45 years), or evidence of the disease in family members. The types 2 and 3 ECG patterns described above are not diagnostic *per se* for Brugada syndrome and require confirmation by additional criteria [3].

The concealed or borderline ECG manifestations of the Brugada syndrome can be unmasked by sodium channel blockers, but also by a febrile state or vagotonic agents. Instead, drug challenge is not performed in patients displaying the type 1 ECG pattern at baseline, because the additional diagnostic value is considered to be limited and the test is not without risk for provoking arrhythmic events.

Recommendations for Sports Participation in Brugada Patients

The Brugada syndrome is associated with risk of SCD due to malignant ventricular arrhythmias (sustained VT, VF), which usually occur at rest and often at night, as a consequence of increased vagal stimulation and/or withdrawal of sympathetic activity. Increased vagal tone as a consequence of chronic athletic conditioning may eventually enhance the propensity of athletes with Brugada syndrome to die at rest, during sleep or during the recovery after exercise. Therefore, although no relation between exercise and arrhythmias has been found, subjects with definite diagnosis of Brugada syndrome should be restricted from competitive sports [5].

Early Repolarization Pattern in Athletes

The ST-segment elevation in trained athletes can be differentiated from ST segment elevation of the Brugada syndrome by its localization and morphology [6]. The most common pattern (type 1, Fig. 15.4a) is characterized by an elevated J point, often associated with notching or slurring of the terminal QRS complex, an upward concavity of the elevated ST-segment and a positive ("peaked and tall") terminal T-wave. Another pattern (type 2) consists of an elevated ST-segment which is convex on the top ("domed") and followed by a negative or small/indistinct T-wave (Fig. 15.4b); this type is most often observed in black people. Early repolarization in trained athletes is usually localized in precordial leads, with the greatest ST-segment elevation in mid-to-lateral leads (V3–V4). Maximal ST-segment displacement may occasionally occur more laterally (leads V5, V6, L1 and aVL), or inferiorly (L2, L3 and aVF).

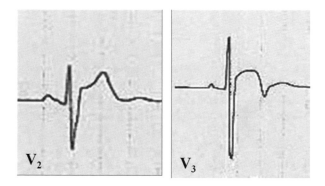

Fig. 15.4a,b The most common ECG patterns of early repolarization in trained athletes. **a** This pattern is characterized by an elevated J point, often associated with notching or slurring of the terminal QRS complex, and an upward concavity of the elevated ST-segment continuing with a positive ("peaked and tall") terminal T-wave. **b** This pattern consists of an elevated ST-segment which is convex on the top ("domed") and followed by a negative or terminal negative T-wave

In our athlete a ST-segment elevation was characterized by a down-sloping pattern evident in lead V2, different from the usual ST-segment elevation with upward concavity and positive T wave seen in most athletes. This ECG pattern raised suspicion for possible expression of the Brugada syndrome and triggered our decision to proceed with provocative testing in order to reliably exclude that diagnosis, and allow athlete to consistently continue his athletic career.

References

1. Pelliccia A, Maron BJ, Culasso F. Clinical significance of abnormal electrocardiographic patterns in trained athletes. Circulation 2000, 102:278–284
2. Brugada P, Brugada J. Right bundle branch block, persistent ST segment elevation and sudden cardiac death: a distinct clinical and electrocardiographic syndrome. J Am Coll Cardiol 1992, 20:1391–1396
3. Antzelevitch C, Brugada P, Borggrefe M. Brugada syndrome: report of the second consensus conference. Circulation 2005, 111:659–670
4. GussaK I, Antzelevitch C, Bjerregaard P. The Brugada syndrome: clinical, electrophysiologic and genetic aspects. J Am Coll Cardiol 1999, 33:5–15
5. Pelliccia A, Fagard R, Bjornstad HH, Anastassakis A, Arbustini E, Assanelli D, Biffi A, Borjesson M, Carre F, Corrado D, Delise P, Dorwarth U, Hirth A, Heidbuchel H, Hoffmann E, Melwig KP, Panhuyzen-Goedkoop NM, Pisani A, Solberg EE, Vanbuuuren F, Vanhees L. Recommendations for competitive sports participation in athletes with cardiovascular disease. Eur Heart J 2005, 26:1422–1445
6. Bianco M, Bria S, Gianfelici A, et al. Does early repolarization in the athlete have analogies with the Brugada syndrome? Eur Heart J 2001, 22:504–510

Chapter 16
A 17-Year-Old Competitive Soccer Player with Pre-excitation Pattern on 12-Lead ECG

Hein Heidbüchel

Family and Personal History

The patient was a 17-year-old soccer player. He played competitive, non-professional, soccer in a regional league, with 1 or 2 matches per week and 2 additional training sessions of 2 h each. He was seen elsewhere for a first screening evaluation. His exercise capacity was unrestricted. There were no familial cases of sudden death or known cardiac disease. He had no special medical history and was fully asymptomatic. Specifically, he never experienced pre-syncope, syncope or paroxysmal palpitations.

Physical Examination

Physical examination was completely normal, with a blood pressure of 136/78 mmHg.

12-Lead ECG

The 12-lead ECG showed pre-excitation pattern (Fig. 16.1). The delta waves were isoelectric in lead V1, positive in lead V2 till V6, and negative in the inferior leads. This pattern indicated a postero-septal location of the accessory pathway [1].

Diagnostic Course

The patient underwent a diagnostic electrophysiological (EP) study, according to the current Recommendations of the ESC [2, 3]. It showed an anterograde refractory periods of the accessory pathway of 270 ms at baseline (under general anesthesia),

H. Heidbüchel (✉)
Department of Cardiology – Electrophysiology, University Hospital Gasthuisberg, University of Leuven, Herestraat 49, B-3000 Leuven, Belgium Europe
e-mail: Hein.Heidbuchel@uz.kuleuven.ac.be

A. Pelliccia (ed.), *Sports Cardiology Casebook*,
DOI 10.1007/978-1-84882-042-5_16, © Springer-Verlag London Limited 2009

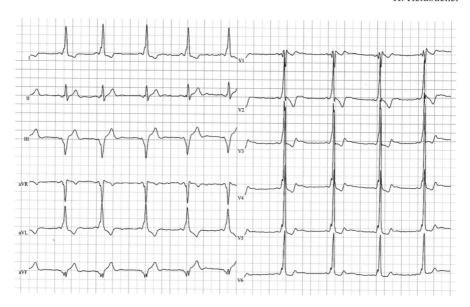

Fig. 16.1 The 12-lead ECG recorded during a preparticipation screening, showing a sinus rhythm at 60 bpm and preexcitation pattern. The delta waves were isoelectric in lead V1, positive in lead V2 till V6, and negative in the inferior leads. This pattern indicated a posteroseptal location of the accessory pathway. This location was eventually confirmed at EP study

decreasing to less than 220 ms during infusion of 0.5 μg/min isoproterenol. Circus movement tachycardia at a rate of 220 bpm could be induced, with anterograde conduction over the AV node and retrograde conduction over the accessory pathway. No atrial fibrillation was induced.

The accessory pathway was located in a right postero-septal position, just outside the ostium of the coronary sinus. It was successfully ablated during the same session with the first application of radiofrequency energy.

Recommendations

The patient was restricted from sport for 1 week and was allowed to resume progressive training from the 2nd week. He could restart competitive sports after 1 month, after a new ECG did not show recurrence of pre-excitation [3].

The athlete underwent further ECG evaluations 6 months and 1 year after ablation, and he continued competitive soccer without restrictions.

Discussion

This case illustrates a typical scenario of a young athlete with asymptomatic preexcitation pattern, occasionally discovered on a pre-participation screening ECG.

The preexcitation is due to abnormal conduction from the atria to the ventricles over an accessory pathway. In such patients, there is a small but definitive risk for sudden death due to development of atrial fibrillation with rapid anterograde conduction over the accessory pathway. Since exercise is associated with an increased risk for sudden death [4], further evaluation is required when an ECG with pre-excitation is recorded during screening in a competitive athlete.

In competitive athletes, EP study is mandatory according to the current Recommendations, to assess the inducibility of tachycardia or atrial fibrillation and to evaluate the shortest pre-excited RR-interval and/or anterograde refractory period [2, 3]. If any of those is ≤ 250 ms, if conduction over the accessory pathway is highly dependent on adrenergic tone (as in this case), or if multiple accessory pathways are present, the athlete-patient is considered at risk and ablation is mandatory.

In individuals participating in leisure-time and amateur sport activities, however, a non-invasive evaluation looking for intermittent pre-excitation on Holter, during an exercise test, or during administration of a low dose class 1 anti-arrhythmic drug might be indicated to assess a low risk situation. Also, in recreational athletes, an invasive study and/or ablation can be considered on an individual basis, weighing risks of ablation vs. potential benefit. Ablation is especially advised for individuals participating in sports with an increased risk due to loss of consciousness (like race pilots, mountain climbing), or those that need a professional license, since it is known that 3.5% of non-inducible patients may become symptomatic during follow-up

Eventually, constraint for invasive procedures is needed in children and young adolescents before the growth spurt. The risk for AF-induced ventricular fibrillation is low at this age and high level competitive sports is rare, and there remains debate on whether the benefits of an aggressive approach outweigh the risks [5–7].

References

1. Arruda MS, McClelland JH, Wang X, Beckman KJ, Wideman LE, Gonzalez MD, Nakagawa H, Lazzara R, Jackman WM. Development and validation of an ECG algorithm for identifying accessory pathway ablation site in Wolff–Parkinson–White syndrome. J Cardiovasc Electrophysiol 1998, 9(1): 2–12
2. Pelliccia A, Fagard R, Bjørnstad HH, Anastassakis A, Arbustini E, Assanelli D, Biffi A, Borjesson M, Carrè F, Corrado D, Delise P, Dorwarth U, Hirth A, Heidbuchel H, Hoffmann E, Mellwig KP, Panhuyzen-Goedkoop N, Pisani A, Solberg E, van-Buuren F, Vanhees L. Recommendations for competitive sports participation in athletes with cardiovascular disease. A Consensus document from the Study Group of Sports Cardiology of the Working Group of Cardiac Rehabilitation and Exercise Physiology, and the Working Group of Myocardial and Pericardial diseases of the European Society of Cardiology. Eur Heart J 2005, 26: 1422–1445
3. Heidbuchel H, Panhuyzen-Goedkoop N, Corrado D, Hoffmann E, Biffi A, Delise P, Blomstrom-Lundqvist C, Vanhees L, Ivarhoff P, Dorwarth U, Pelliccia A. Recommendations for participation in leisure-time physical activity and competitive sports in patients with arrhythmias and potentially arrhythmogenic conditions Part I: Supraventricular arrhythmias and pacemakers. Eur J Cardiovasc Prev Rehabil Aug 2006, 13(4):475–484
4. Timmermans C, Smeets JL, Rodriguez LM, Vrouchos G, van den Dool A, Wellens HJ. Aborted sudden death in the Wolff-Parkinson-White syndrome. Am J Cardiol Sep 1 1995, 76(7): 492–494

5. Delise P, Sciarra L. Asymptomatic Wolff-Parkinson-White: what to do. Extensive ablation or not? J Cardiovasc Med (Hagerstown) Sep 2007, 8(9):668–674
6. Wellens HJ. Should catheter ablation be performed in asymptomatic patients with Wolff-Parkinson-White syndrome? When to perform catheter ablation in asymptomatic patients with a Wolff-Parkinson-White electrocardiogram. Circulation Oct 4 2005, 112(14):2201–2207; discussion 2216
7. Pappone C, Santinelli V, Manguso F, Augello G, Santinelli O, Vicedomini G, Gulletta S, Mazzone P, Tortoriello V, Pappone A, Dicandia C, Rosanio S. A randomized study of prophylactic catheter ablation in asymptomatic patients with the Wolff-Parkinson-White syndrome. N Engl J Med Nov 6 2003, 349(19):1803–1811

Chapter 17
A Symptomatic Judoka with Wolff-Parkinson-White Pattern

Mohamed Tahmi

Athletic History

This is a 18-year-old high-level male judoka. He has been practicing judo since he was 13 years old. In the last 3 years his training schedule was up to 18 h per week. At present he competes at national level.

Family History

His familial history reveals no known congenital or other cardiovascular diseases and no known cases of premature (<50 years) sudden cardiac death among close relatives.

Personal History

The onset of clinical history was at age of 14 years (March 2003). He had prolonged and rapid palpitations which emerged abruptly during sports activity, recognized on 12-lead ECG as atrial fibrillation and required an electric shock. The ECG recorded at that time showed preexcitation pattern, i.e., Wolff-Parkinson-White (WPW) syndrome. After that initial episode, he was considered ineligible for competitive sports activity and treatment with amiodarone (400 mg daily) was prescribed.

Physical Examination

The physical examination showed normal findings on heart and lung auscultation.In particular, no valvular disease was found. The resting heart rate was 70 bpm. The blood pressure was 120/80 mmHg.

M. Tahmi (✉)
Department of Cardiology, CHU Tizi Ouzou, Nédir Hospital-Tizi-Ouzou University, Tizi-Ouzou, Algeria
e-mail: mtahmi@hotmail.com

A. Pelliccia (ed.), *Sports Cardiology Casebook*,
DOI 10.1007/978-1-84882-042-5_17, © Springer-Verlag London Limited 2009

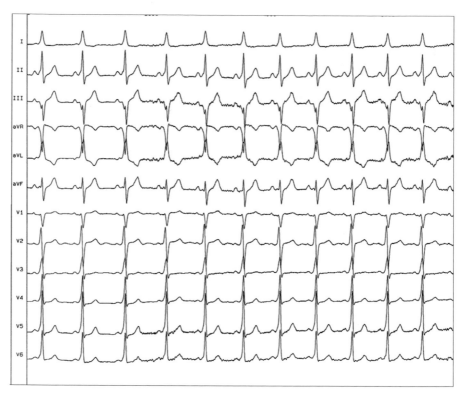

Fig. 17.1 The baseline 12-lead ECG shows preexcitation consistent with localisation of the Kent bundle in right posterior and interventricular septum

12-Lead ECG

A sinus rhythm was observed. A short PR interval and delta wave were evident and the overall pattern was consistent with preexcitation with localisation of the Kent bundle in right posterior and interventricular septum (Fig. 17.1).

Echocardiography

Resting transthoracic echocardiography was considered as normal. No associated structural disease, such as hypertrophic cardiomyopathy, Ebstein anomaly or valvular disease were noted.

Electrophysiologic Study and Ablation Procedure

The patient was referred for ablation of the accessory pathway. In fact, given the history of rapid AF with preexcitation, this athlete was considered to be at risk and indication for ablation was done. During the EP study, atrial fibrillation was easily

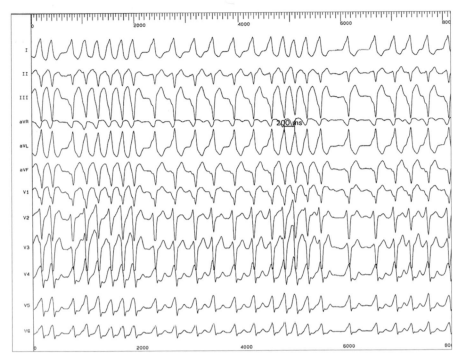

Fig. 17.2 Per-electrophysiology session atrial fibrillation induced, with the shortest RR interval duration measured (200 ms)

induced, with a shortest RR interval of 200 ms (Fig. 17.2). Atrial fibrillation was converted and a successful catheter ablation of the Kent bundle was then performed (Fig. 17.3).

Clinical Course and Recommendations

The clinical course after ablation was without complications: the athlete had no recurrence of symptoms and especially no palpitations or irregular heart beats. The 12-lead ECG pattern remained normal. In accordance with the Bethesda and ESC recommendations he was authorized to resume competitive sports three months post ablation. Serial ECG recordings performed after 6 months remained normal. At present, the athlete continues his competitive sport activity without symptoms or any performance limitation.

Discussion

The prevalence of preexcitation is similar (0.1–0.3%) in athletic and general populations. Atrial fibrillation or atrial flutter may cause rapid activation of the ventricles through the accessory pathway and degenerate into ventricular fibrillation and

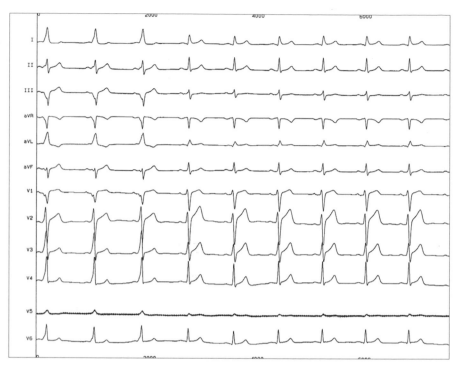

Fig. 17.3 Radiofrequency ablation procedure with transition from WPW pattern to normal AV conduction

sudden cardiac death. The overall risk for sudden cardiac in WPW patients (due to ventricular fibrillation) is quite low and ranges from 0.1% to 0.2%, but appears to be higher (2.2%) in symptomatic patients. This was also the case of our athlete, who experienced rapid fibrillation requiring DC shock. Symptomatic athletes with WPW syndrome and documented arrhythmias, such as atrial fibrillation, should be treated with radiofrequency ablation of the accessory pathway. This was the case of our athlete, who had documented spontaneous atrial fibrillation and, in addition, showed short RR interval of the pre-excited beats during induced atrial fibrillation. In the absence of such a clinical history, risk assessment in competitive athletes with preexcitation should be based on an electrophysiologic study, including measurement of refractoriness of the accessory pathway and induction of atrial fibrillation to assess the shortest pre-excited RR interval. A short pre-excited RR interval (≤240 ms during induced atrial fibrillation and ≤220 ms during effort or isoproterenol infusion), the presence of multiple accessory pathways, and/or easy induction of atrial fibrillation are considered to be associated with an increased risk [1, 2].

In case of asymptomatic athlete with preexcitation and with increased risk as previously specified, ablation is mandatory, both in competitive and leisure time athletes [2]. After catheter ablation, if no recurrence and no cardiac disease, all competitive sports can be resumed. The time to resume competitions should be individualised (depending on prior history, risk stratification and ease of ablation). Resumption of light to moderate training activities is usually possible after 2 weeks, but competition should in many cases be prudently postponed for between 1 and 3 months [2].

References

1. Pelliccia A, Fagard R, Bjørnstad HH, Anastassakis A, Arbustini E, Assanelli D, Biffi A, Borjesson M, Carrè F, Corrado D, Delise P, Dorwarth U, Hirth A, Heidbuchel H, Hoffmann E, Mellwig KP, Panhuyzen-Goedkoop N, Pisani A, Solberg E, van-Buuren F, Vanhees L. Recommendations for competitive sports participation in athletes with cardiovascular disease. A Consensus document from the Study Group of Sports Cardiology of the Working Group of Cardiac Rehabilitation and Exercise Physiology, and the Working Group of Myocardial and Pericardial Diseases of the European Society of Cardiology. Eur Heart J 2005, 26: 1422–1445
2. Heidbuchel H, Panhuyzen-Goedkoop N, Corrado D, Hoffmann, H, Biffi A, Delise P, Blomstrom-Lundqvist C, Vanhees L, Ivarhoff P, Dorwath U, Pelliccia A. Recommendations for participation in leisure-time physical activity and competitive sports in patients with arrhythmias and potentially arrhythmogenic conditions. Part I : Supraventricular arrhythmias and pacemakers. Eur J Prev Cardiovasc Rehabil 2006, 13: 475–484

Chapter 18
A 35-Year-Old Competitive Cyclist with Frequent Premature Ventricular Beats

Hein Heidbüchel

Athlete's History

The patient was a 35-year-old competitive but non-professional cyclist. He started competitive cycling during his teenage years and was still continuing this activity until the date of evaluation. At the top of his athletic career, he competed on a national level, with an average of 1 to 2 races per week and daily training of a 3–4 hours(h).

Previous Diagnostic Testing

He underwent a routine cardiologic check-up elsewhere 1 year ago. The ECG recorded at that time is shown in Fig. 18.1. It revealed a sinus rhythm at 60 bpm with two isolated premature ventricular beats (PVB) with a right bundle branch block morphology and superior axis. The sinus rhythm QRS had a right axis deviation and there were diffuse negative T-waves in the left precordial leads V_4 to V_6 and standard leads II, III and aVF. An ECG Holter monitoring was performed at that time which showed more than 5,000 PVBs per 24 h, all monomorphic. During exercise test, the frequency of PVBs decreased. Echocardiography was normal. Given the fact that the athlete was fully asymptomatic and the ECG findings were considered non-diagnostic for pathologic cardiac condition, the athlete was allowed resumption of competitive sport.

Medical History

After about 1 year, the athlete presented complaining of dyspnoea during exercise, described as "fast, uncontrolled respiration" accompanied with slight dizziness. The

H. Heidbüchel (✉)
Department of Cardiology – Electrophysiology, University Hospital Gasthuisberg, University of Leuven, Herestraat 49, B-3000 Leuven, Belgium Europe
e-mail: hein.heidbuchel@uz.kuleuven.ac.be

A. Pelliccia (ed.), *Sports Cardiology Casebook*,
DOI 10.1007/978-1-84882-042-5_18, © Springer-Verlag London Limited 2009

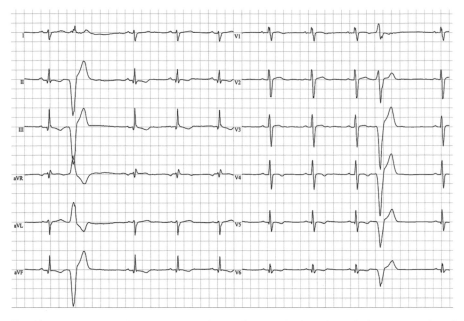

Fig. 18.1 The 12-lead ECG during a routine cardiologic check-up 1 year before presentation of symptoms. The ECG showed a sinus rhythm at 60 bpm with two isolated ventricular premature beats (with a right bundle branch block morphology and superior axis). The sinus rhythm QRS had a right axis deviation and there were negative T-waves in the left precordial leads V_4 to V_6 and standard leads II, III and aVF

athlete did not report palpitations, no pre-syncope and he never developed syncope. He underwent a respiratory evaluation, which included a normal spirometry, and negative hyperventilation and histamine provocation test. He was referred, therefore, to our Institute for a second opinion.

Physical Examination

The physical examination was unremarkable.

12-Lead ECG

The 12-lead ECG revealed a sinus rhythm at 50 bpm, with right axis deviation and with diffusely inverted T-waves as shown in the ECG 1 year before, but without ventricular premature beats (Fig. 18.2).

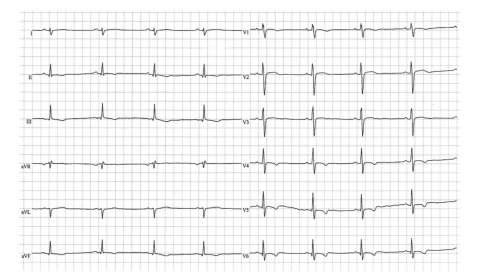

Fig. 18.2 A 12-lead ECG at initial presentation in our Institute with a sinus rhythm of 50 bpm and without ventricular ectopic beats. The right axis deviation and diffusely inverted T-waves were present as one year before

New Diagnostic Testing

A new Holter monitoring showed 2,200 PVBs per 24 h and sporadic couplets. Exercise testing led to the induction of isolated PVBs above 50 W (Fig. 18.3). The repolarization abnormalities remained substantially unchanged. At a load of 275 W,

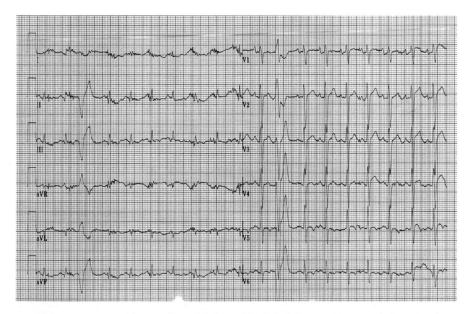

Fig. 18.3 Exercise testing led to the induction of isolated VPBs at loads above 50 W (here shown at 175 W)

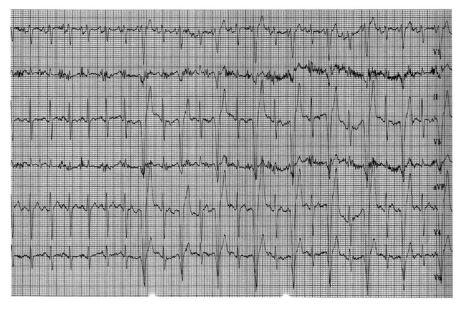

Fig. 18.4 ECG at 275 W during an exercise test, showing an episode of monomorphic VPB in bigeminy

bigeminy PVBs developed for a short time period (Fig. 18.4). The maximal exercise level was 375 W, with a progressive decrease and finally disappearance of PVBs above loads of 275 W. The patient developed a blood pressure drop after exercising (from 210/90 mmHg to 150/60 mmHg, continuous sinus rhythm), which was associated with dizziness resembling his clinical symptoms. Echocardiography showed mildly dilated right and left ventricles with normal function, which were considered to be consistent with athlete's heart. Cardiac Magnetic Resonance (CMR) was performed, which showed a normal right and left ventricle, without fatty infiltration and without regional wall motion abnormalities in either ventricle.

Since this observation did not explain completely the patient's symptoms induced by exercise, a further diagnostic evaluation was programmed. Coronary angiogram was performed, which showed normal LV morphology with global ejection fraction of 69% and no evident regional wall motion abnormalities, except a suspicion for mild hypokinesia over the antero-lateral wall. Right ventricular (RV) angiography showed a mildly dilated and hypokinetic chamber, which was interpreted visually as athlete's heart. However, quantitative RV ejection fraction assessment, using specified algorithms and software, showed mildly decreased ejection fraction of 49% (Fig. 18.5) [1].

A late potential ECG revealed 2 out of 3 positive criteria: filtered QRS duration 133 ms and HFLA duration 41 ms (Fig. 18.6), while RMS40 was normal (24μV). Electrophysiologic (EP) study was performed, which induced three different forms of sustained monomorphic VT, with rates between 195 and 250 bpm, all with a left

Fig. 18.5 End-diastolic (**top**) and end-systolic (**bottom**) frames of RV angiography (RAO projections in left column, LAO at right side). Quantitative RV ejection fraction determination using specified algorithms and software calculated a mildly decreased fraction of 49% RV ejection, although the angiography was visually (qualitatively) judged to be within normal limits for athlete's heart

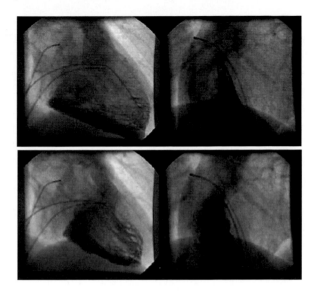

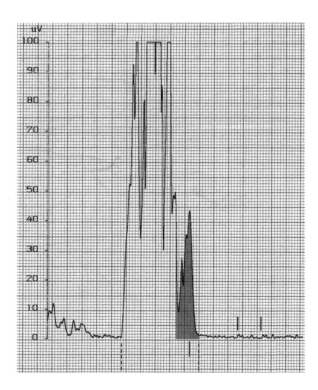

Fig. 18.6 Two out of three criteria were positive for late potentials: filtered QRS duration 134 ms (normal ≤120 ms); duration of the high-frequency low-amplitude signals ≤40 μV (HFLA40) 41 ms (normal <40 ms). Root mean square voltage of the last 40 ms (RMS40) was 24 μV (normal >20 μV)

bundle branch block morphology. Each morphology was different from the morphology of the isolated PVB observed on the baseline ECG and exercise tests.

Recommendations and Treatment

The patient was advised to stop any competitive and intensive sports activity [2]. Beta-blockers were started at a low dose, which were well tolerated. The patient was eventually advised of the opportunity for prophylactic ICD implantation. The patient agreed and an ICD was implanted.

Clinical Course

One year later he developed a first ICD intervention (Fig. 18.7). A shock was delivered for a fast regular ventricular tachycardia at 220 bpm, which developed while the patient was watching a cycling event and which was associated with dizziness.

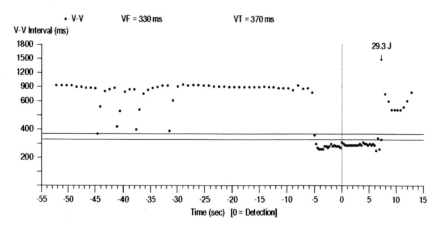

Fig. 18.7 One year after ICD implantation, the athlete received a first shock. The figure shows the interval plot of a fast ventricular tachycardia (220 bpm) that developed while watching a cycling event. The first 30 J shock restored sinus rhythm. The patient felt short dizziness before the shock

Discussion

This case illustrates the importance of a comprehensive cardiologic evaluation when a patient reports exercise-related symptoms, such as dyspnoea in this case. Although originally a respiratory origin of symptoms was suspected, the arrhythmic aetiology was considered and fully evaluated. The case even illustrates that a more scrupulous cardiologic evaluation might have been appropriate already 1 year earlier, when the ECG showed diffusely inverted T-waves and PVBs, although the patient was still asymptomatic.

The ECG Holter monitoring had shown more than 2.000 PVBs per 24 h. Prior studies have revealed 30% risk of underlying cardiac abnormality when frequent ventricular ectopy is found on a Holter monitoring [3]. The athlete also had positive late potentials, a non-invasive test which could have indicated probable underlying structural abnormality. However, imaging techniques did not reveal striking abnormalities. Only quantitative evaluation of RV ejection fraction (which is not still implemented in the routine clinical practice) showed a slightly subnormal value. Recent evidence has shown that athletes with ventricular arrhythmias originating from the right ventricle and mildly decreased RV ejection fraction are likely to represent expression of underlying RV cardiomyopathy. Quantitative evaluation of the RV function is not part so far of the diagnostic algorithm for ARVC [4], but may be of particular relevance in an athletic population [1]. The classic criteria for ARVC were not diagnostic for the disease in this athlete (three minor criteria were present). This occurrence is not rare in the athlete population, since morphologic expression of the disease may be concealed for a period before complete clinical picture become evident (and diagnosis according to the task force criteria definite).

A genetic testing for sequencing of five desmosomal genes was performed, but revealed no mutation. The aetiology of the underlying structural abnormality in this athlete therefore remained elusive. This case also illustrates the potential value of performing an invasive EP study in an athlete with exercise-related symptoms and suspicion of underlying structural abnormalities [5]. The EP study showed induction of multiple re-entrant arrhythmic circuits of RV origin. There is no prospective data on the best management in such cases, i.e. whether termination of competitive sports, combined with beta-blockers or other anti-arrhythmic treatment suffices to prevent further life-threatening arrhythmias, or whether ICD implantation should be recommended.

In this case it is likely that ICD implantation has prevented potentially life-threatening tachyarrhythmia. It is important to note that the patient had effectively stopped his competitive sports and also did not participate anymore to any intense recreational activities. He also had continued to take his beta-blockers. The arrhythmia terminated by the ICD discharge developed not during exercise but during an emotional period while he was watching a cycling event.

In conclusion, this case clearly demonstrates the need for thorough and individualised cardiovascular evaluation in an athlete with PVBs and symptoms, even if the initial presentation was one with only apparently innocent PVBs.

References

1. Ector J, Ganame J, van der Merwe N, Adriaenssens B, Pison L, Willems R, Gewillig M, Heidbuchel H. Reduced right ventricular ejection fraction in endurance athletes presenting with ventricular arrhythmias: a quantitative angiographic assessment. Eur Heart J 2007, 28:345–353
2. Heidbuchel H, Corrado D, Biffi A, Hoffmann E, Panhuyzen-Goedkoop N, Hoogsteen J, Delise P, Hoff PI, Pelliccia A. Recommendations for participation in leisure-time physical activity and competitive sports of patients with arrhythmias and potentially arrhythmogenic conditions. Part II: Ventricular arrhythmias, channelopathies and implantable defibrillators. Eur J Cardiovasc Prev Rehabil 2006,13:676–686
3. Biffi A, Pelliccia A, Verdile L, Fernando F, Spataro A, Caselli S, Santini M, Maron BJ. Long-term clinical significance of frequent and complex ventricular tachyarrhythmias in trained athletes. J Am Coll Cardiol Aug 7 2002, 40:446–452
4. McKenna WJ, Thiene G, Nava A, Fontaliran F, Blomstrom Lundqvist C, Fontaine G, Camerini F. Diagnosis of arrhythmogenic right ventricular dysplasia/cardiomyopathy. Task Force of the Working Group Myocardial and Pericardial Disease of the European Society of Cardiology and of the Scientific Council on Cardiomyopathies of the International Society and Federation of Cardiology. Br Heart J 1994, 71:215–218
5. Heidbuchel H, Hoogsteen J, Fagard R, Vanhees L, Ector H, Willems R, Van Lierde J. High prevalence of right ventricular involvement in endurance athletes with ventricular arrhythmias. Role of an electrophysiologic study in risk stratification. Eur Heart J 2003, 24:1473–1480

Chapter 19
An Athlete with Ischemic Pattern on Exercise ECG

Elvira DeBlasiis, Fernando Maria Di Paolo, and Antonio Pelliccia

Family and Personal History

This is a 28-year-old, male athlete who was selected in 2003 as a member of the Italian National Rowing Team because of his excellent athletic achievements. Personal history was negative for CV diseases or any cardiac symptoms. He was a non-smoker and he denied use of drugs or medicaments. Family history was positive for systemic hypertension and diabetes, but no history of ischemic heart disease or premature sudden death was reported in close relatives.

Physical Examination

The athlete was in a good shape and excellent athletic condition; weight was 74 kg, height 176 cm, with a BSA of 1.9 m^2. On cardiovascular physical examination, the blood pressure was 140/70 mmHg, and there were no murmurs or abnormal heart sounds.

12-Lead ECG

The 12-lead ECG showed sinus bradycardia (55 bpm) with normal QRS axis, and 1st degree AV block (PR interval: 0.23 s). QTc interval was within normal limits (0.44 s). The R/S wave voltages were mildly increased in precordial leads V5, V6, and repolarization pattern was normal (Fig. 19.1).

E. DeBlasiis (✉)
Institute of Sports Medicine and Science, Italian National Olympic Committee, Department of Sport Medicine, Largo Piero Gabrielli, 1 00197 Rome, Italy
e-mail: elvdeb@tin.it

A. Pelliccia (ed.), *Sports Cardiology Casebook*,
DOI 10.1007/978-1-84882-042-5_19, © Springer-Verlag London Limited 2009

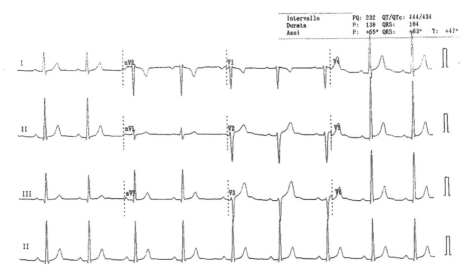

Fig. 19.1 Baseline 12-lead ECG. Sinus bradycardia (54 bpm) with normal axis, 1st AV block (PR interval: 0.23 s). and QTc interval within normal limits (0.44 s) were evident. The R/S wave voltages were mildly increased in precordial leads V4, V5, and repolarization pattern was normal

Exercise Electrocardiography

On exercise testing, starting from 50 W for 2 min, with increments of 50 W every 2 min, he reached 350 W, with a maximum heart rate of 182 bpm and blood pressure of 230/70 mmHg. During exercise, a progressive downsloping depression of the ST-segment in precordial leads from V4 to V6 was observed, which was ≥3 mm at peak exercise, and associated with inversion of T wave in same leads, in the absence of symptoms (Fig. 19.2). In addition, monomorphic premature ventricular beats (PVBs), with left bundle branch block (LBBB) morphology were observed.

Echocardiography

The echocardiographic study showed the origin of left main and right coronary artery in the normal position (Fig. 19.3). Indeed, the study showed the typical left ventricular (LV) remodeling of athlete's heart. The LV cavity was enlarged (end-diastolic diameter = 58 mm), ventricular septum and free wall were at upper normal limits (11 mm), there was no evidence of segmental hypertrophy and the overall picture did not suggest hypertrophic cardiomyopathy. LV global systolic function was normal (EF 63%) in the absence of wall motion abnormalities, and so was the diastolic filling and relaxation pattern, as assessed by transmitral Doppler and Tissue Doppler Imaging, respectively. The left atrium was at upper normal limits

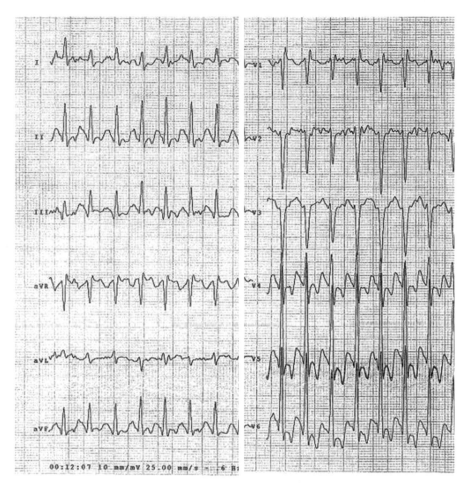

Fig. 19.2 Electrocardiogram recorded during exercise testing. Significant downsloping of the ST segment, up to 3 mm at peak exercise, is present in precordial leads V4 to V6, associated with of T-wave inversion

(transverse diameter = 40 mm). The right ventricle did not show any morphologic or functional abnormality.

ECG Holter Monitoring

In order to evaluate the severity of ventricular arrhythmia, an ECG Holter monitoring was performed, including a session of physical training. This testing showed only a rare ventricular arrhythmia (i.e., 54 PVBs with LBBB morphology in 24 h), and confirmed the presence of 1st AV block (PR interval 0.23 s), which disappeared during effort.

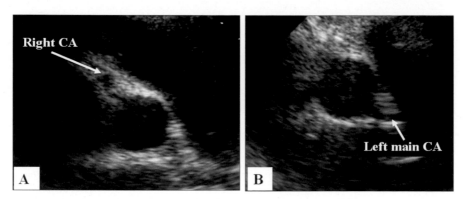

Fig. 19.3a,b Echocardiographic study showing the origin of left main and right coronary artery. **a** Right coronary artery ostium and proximal course. **b** Left main coronary artery ostium and proximal course

Other Tests

Blood count showed a mild anemia (Hb 13.7 g/dL, Ht 39%). The total cholesterol was 195 mg/dL, LDL 153 mg/dL and HDL 50 mg/dL.

Ventriculo-Coronary Angiography

To assess the possible ischemic significance of the abnormal ECG pattern observed during exercise further diagnostic testing were planned and the athlete was temporarily withdrawn from competitions. The athlete underwent ventriculo-coronary angiography which confirmed the normal position of both ostia of coronary arteries and the normal proximal course, with a right dominance. No significant atherosclerotic lesions were found along the coronary vessels. Separated origin of the ramus coronalis was described (Video 19.1). Left ventricle was mildly enlarged with normal systolic function and diastolic filling. No morphologic abnormalities were described in the right ventricle.

Video 19.1a–c Coronary angiography showing the normal position of coronary arteries ostia and course with a right dominance, in the absence of any atherosclerotic lesion or intramural course (myocardial bridge). **a,b** Left coronary artery. **c** Right coronary artery

Cardiac Magnetic Resonance

In addition, cardiac magnetic resonance (CMR) was performed. LV morphology was normal (with mild enlargement of LV cavity), systolic function and contractility were normal. The right ventricular cavity was normal with the presence of a prominent apical trabeculations. Delayed enhancement with post-gadolinium showed no alterations in the signal and no fat infiltration in the right ventricle.

Diagnosis and Recommendations

The athlete was considered free of coronary artery and myocardial disease and no restriction were applied for him to participate in training and competitions.

In the subsequent 5-year follow-up, the athlete had periodical cardiac evaluations in our Institute; the abnormal ECG pattern induced by exercise has remained substantially unchanged until present time. In the same period, he did not report symptoms nor cardiac events.

Discussion

The most striking abnormality found in this athlete was the substantial repolarization abnormality (i.e., significant downsloping depression of the ST-segment) induced by exercise, which was instinctively suggestive for ischemic heart disease. In consideration of the young age of the subject and the low risk profile, the hypothesis considered most probable was the presence of a congenital coronary artery anomaly, such as an abnormal origin and/or proximal course (i.e., myocardial bridging). Therefore, imaging testing were required to solve this question; the echocardiography showed a normal position of both the coronary ostia. The echocardiography is usually capable to visualize the origin and proximal course of the coronary artery in a large proportion of young individuals (in our athlete population, the ostium of the left main coronary artery is imaged in >95% of athletes and that of the right coronary artery in >80%) [1]. The information derived from this testing were, in fact, confirmed by the subsequent ventriculo-coronary angiography. Another possibility was the presence of intramural coronary artery course. Presence of myocardial bridge is not uncommon in asymptomatic individuals and represents an occasional finding in about 5% of autopsies [2]. The clinical significance of myocardial bridge is unresolved, but this abnormality has been described in selected individuals who have died suddenly, in particular in young subjects with hypertrophic cardiomyopathy [3]. For this reason, we were ethically and legally forced to exclude this abnormality in our athlete. Therefore, he underwent ventriculo-coronary angiography, which excluded such abnormality and, indeed, any significant atherosclerotic lesion.

Occurrence of an abnormal repolarization pattern induced by exercise testing, mimicking myocardial ischemia, has been reported in a substantial minority of young individuals (including athletes) without evidence of cardiovascular disease, namely ischemic heart disease [4]. Mechanisms producing such markedly abnormal pattern during exercise remained unknown. As possible explanation, imbalance between the sympathetic and parasympathetic activity of the autonomic nervous system can be advocated [5]; specifically, it has been supposed that the increased sympathetic drive during exercise may increase the myocardial oxygen consumption in selected individuals up to overcome the coronary blood flow and mimicking an ischemic ECG pattern. The clinical significance of such abnormal ECG response to exercise appears to be benign and, although long-term observation is required, our case suggests that no symptoms or events occurred in a medium-term follow-up.

References

1. Pelliccia A, Spataro A, Maron BJ. Prospective echocardiographic screening for coronary artery anomalies in 1,360 elite competitive athletes. Am J Cardiol 1993, 15(72):978–979
2. Morales AR, Romanelli R, Boucek RJ. The mural left anterior descending coronary artery, strenuous exercise and sudden death. Circulation 1980, 62:230–237
3. Yetman AT, McCrindle BW, et al. Myocardial bridging in children with hypertrophic cardiomyopathy – a risk factor for sudden death. N Engl J Med 1998, 22(339):1201–1209
4. Spirito P, Maron BJ, et al. Prevalence and significance of an abnormal S-T segment response to exercise in a young athletic population. Am J Cardiol 1993, 51:1663–1666
5. Taggard P, Donaldson R, Green J, et al. Interrelation of heart rate and autonomic activity in asymptomatic men with unobstructed coronary arteries. Br Heart J 1982, 47:19

Chapter 20
A 17-Year-Old National Cyclist with Exercise-Induced Ventricular Tachycardia

Axel J.P. Urhausen, Charles Delagardelle, Camille Pesch, and Hein Heidbüchel

Family and Personal History

The patient is a 17-year-old male athlete in apparently good health. In the last 5 years he was engaged in competitive cycling by training for about 20–25 hours (h) per week, and achieved a national and international level. He was recently selected as member of the junior national team. Since a head trauma in early childhood he showed a nystagmus. No previous cardiac disease or known cardiovascular risk factors were present. The patient was free of medications and denied the intake of doping substances. Also his father and grandfather were internationally successful competitive cyclists. His close relatives had no known cases of premature (<50 years) sudden cardiac death. His grandfather underwent coronary revascularization at the age of 67 and a pacemaker implantation at 73 years.

Medical History

Five months before the beginning of symptoms the athlete had a routine annual sports medical examination including a 12-lead ECG at rest, incremental maximal exercise testing (reaching 350 W, with a peak heart rate of 205 bpm) and echocardiography. These examinations were normal. The medical history started with occurrence of palpitations, thoracic oppression, effort dyspnoea and loss of power during high-intensity competition. These symptoms had started approximately 2 months before our evaluation. Self-monitored heart rate recordings during races showed episodes of heart rates up to 220–230 bpm at those instances (Fig. 20.1).

A.J.P. Urhausen (✉)
Service de Médecine du Sport et de Prévention, Centre de l' Appareil Locomoteur, de Médecine du Sport et de Prévention, Centre Hospitalier de Luxembourg-Clinique d'Eich, Luxembourg
e-mail: urhausen.axel@chl.lu

A. Pelliccia (ed.), *Sports Cardiology Casebook*,
DOI 10.1007/978-1-84882-042-5_20, © Springer-Verlag London Limited 2009

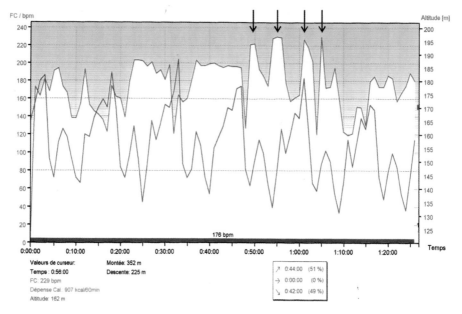

Fig. 20.1 Self-recorded heart rate profile (*upper red line*) and altitude (*lower red line*) during cycling race showing four bouts of heart rate >220 bpm (see *arrows*), not all related to climbing a hill

Physical Examination

The physical examination showed normal heart and lung auscultation. The resting pulse was 51 bpm and the blood pressure 100/60 mmHg.

12-Lead ECG

The 12-lead ECG showed a T-wave inversion in V_2 and a pattern of early repolarization; Overall the pattern was considered to be within normal limits (Fig. 20.2).

Echocardiography

The morphologic features were judged to be consistent with an "athlete's heart", with a total heart volume of 1075 mL (15.5 mL per kg body mass), a left ventricular (LV) mass of 137 g per m² body surface area, LV end-diastolic/systolic diameters of 57 respectively 38 mm, LV wall thickness of 11 mm and a left atrium of 39 mm. Systolic (EF 60%) and diastolic LV function (E/A ratio >1), valves morphology and pericardium were normal.

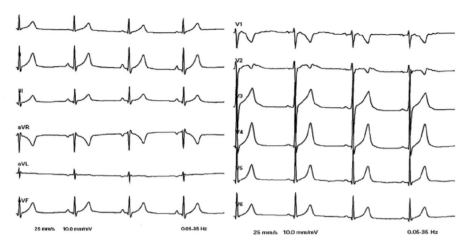

Fig. 20.2 12-lead ECG at baseline, which was described as normal, with possible exception of the negative T-waves in precordial lead V_2

Blood Analysis

Normal findings including CRP, CPK and TSH.

Exercise Test: Race Simulation

A 1-h exercise test simulating competition with high-intensive intervals was performed in the laboratory on his own bike. The ECG remained normal until a heart rate of 199 bpm. At heart rates >200 bpm isolated supraventricular premature beats (SVPBs) appeared and also monomorphic premature ventricular beats (PVBs) with a left bundle branch block configuration. When the exercise reached high workload, PVBs increased further, resulting in ventricular quadri-, tri- and finally bigeminy rhythms (Fig. 20.3). There was no induction of ventricular tachycardia.

Holter ECG Monitoring During Bicycle Race

As a consequence of the exercise testing, ECG Holter monitoring was performed during a real bicycle race. Several episodes of monomorphic sustained ventricular tachycardia (VT) with heart rates of 200−260 bpm were recorded, also lasting several minutes (Fig. 20.4). They were associated with the same clinical symptoms reported in the history.

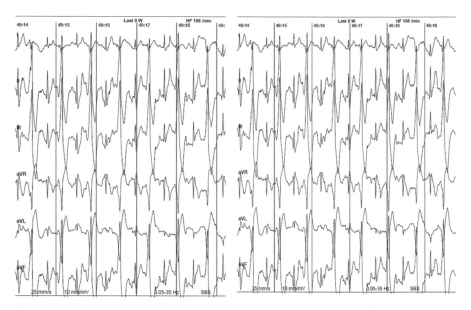

Fig. 20.3 Ventricular bigeminus rhythm during 1-h race simulation with exercise testing in the laboratory

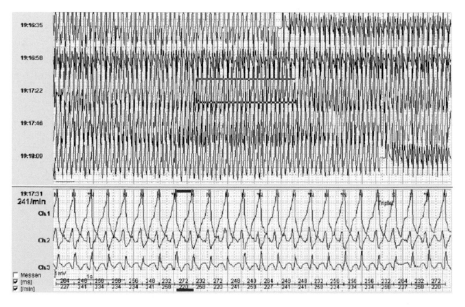

Fig. 20.4 ECG Holter monitoring during a cycling road race revealing ventricular tachycardia of 241 bpm

Recommendations

Due to the appearance of sustained VT and associated symptoms, the athlete was restricted from competition [1, 2] and advised further diagnostic testing in order to exclude underlying structural disease, find out the VT origin and possibly to initiate specific treatment.

Additional Diagnostic Tests

Coronary-angiography (no significant coronary lesions) and cardiac magnetic resonance (no left ventricular wall thickening, no wall motion abnormalities, normal right ventricular size and function) were normal.

Electrophysiologic Study

Two electrophysiologic studies were performed in the subsequent period. There was no evidence of pre-excitation. Both EP studies were unable to induce VT despite programmed stimulation with up to three extrastimuli at the apex and at the RVOT, either at baseline and during infusion of isoproterenol (with increasing dose until a heart rate of 160 bpm) and atropine (0.5 mg). During isoproterenol infusion, however, spontaneous isolated PVBs from the RVOT were recorded.

Mapping was difficult because of the rare PVBs. Pace mapping at RVOT never succeeded in obtaining a clear and complete match of the stimulated QRS morphology with the spontaneous VTs. Two unsuccessful attempts of ablation were made. The morphology of the PVBs (with rS in peripheral lead I and transition between precordial leads V2 and V3) was suggestive of a location of the arrhythmic focus within the aortic cusp.

Subsequent Clinical Course

In the subsequent months several follow-up investigations were performed:

– A laboratory simulation of high-intense training with heart rate >200 bpm induced only few monomorphic PVBs (quadrigeminus) after exercise
– However, ECG Holter monitoring during a road cycling competition confirmed the occurrence of the same symptoms and several bouts of VT

The patient was therefore referred to another specialized medical center where a third electrophysiologic study was performed. The arrhythmogenic focus was mapped to the LVOT, near the left coronary cusp of the aortic valve. A new ablation attempt was performed which was eventually successful in abolishing the VT focus.

Continued Follow-Up

After that procedure, the athlete remained asymptomatic. Two months later a new maximal exercise test was performed: 400 W (with a heart rate of 203 bpm) was reached, without induction of PVBs nor symptoms.

A new ECG Holter monitoring during strength training, followed by intense cycling training showed only four PVBs and a few SVPBs, without any subjective complaints.

In the following months four more ECG Holter monitoring recordinges were performed during cycling races (maximal heart rate of 200–210 bpm) which all remained negative. At that time, in consideration of the proven success of the ablation, the absence of symptoms and failure to induce VTs, the athlete was allowed to resume full competitive activity.

After 18 months, he is still without subjective complaints and has very good competitive performances (national level). No arrhythmias were induced during subsequent maximal exercise testing, nor recorded by ECG Holter monitoring during competition. No morphologic or functional abnormalities were found in subsequent echocardiographic investigations.

Final Recommendations

Cycling is listed in the Bethesda Classification as a very high dynamic and very high static sport, thus involving maximal cardiovascular strain [1]. In accordance with the current European recommendations [2, 3], the athlete has been finally declared eligible for competitive cycling in consideration of the documented absence of any significant ventricular arrhythmias during training and competition, the absence of structural heart disease, and total regression of symptoms after successful ablation. However, a periodical follow-up testing is required, including maximal exercise testing, echocardiography and ECG Holter monitoring (including cycling race) every 12 months, to exclude progression of any underlying structural or arrhythmogenic condition.

Discussion

Ergometric tests performed to exclude cardiac abnormalities in competitive athletes should be conducted until maximal exhaustion. Even by doing so, the actual cardiac strain of competition is not always reached, especially in cycling, a sport with very high dynamic and static demands over a long time. In the present case even aggressive stimulation protocols in several electrophysiologic studies only induced isolated PVBs. In a race simulation, on the personal competition bike of the athlete in the laboratory, a maximal heart rate >200 bpm was reached. However, only PVBs – ventricular quadri-, tri- and finally bigeminy – could be induced. Both lab tests were not able to provoke the same bouts of sustained VT that appeared on Holter monitoring only during a real race.

This example also supports the usefulness of regular cardiac examinations in competitive athletes, which should include an exercise ECG, at least in sports with higher cardiovascular demands. These exams not only help to minimize the probability of the existence of a underlying disease but it also allows a comparison with previous values in case of occurrence of new complaints.

References

1. Mitchell JH, Haskell WL, Snell P, Van Camp SP (2005) Task Force 8: classification of sports. J Am Coll Cardiol 45:1364–1367
2. Pelliccia A, Fagard R, Bjørnstad HH, Anastassakis A, Arbustini E, Assanelli D, Biffi A, Borjesson M, Carré F, Corrado D, Delise P, Dorwarth U, Hirth A, Heidbuchel H, Hoffmann E, Mellwig KP, Panhuyzen-Goedkoop N, Pisani A, Solberg EE, van-Buuren F, Vanhees L (2005) Recommendations for competitive sports participation in athletes with cardiovascular disease. A consensus document from the Study Group of Sports Cardiology of the Working Group of Cardiac Rehabilitation and Exercise Physiology and the Working Group of Myocardial and Pericardial Diseases of the European Society of Cardiology. Eur Heart J 26:1422–1445
3. Heidbuchel H, Corrado D, Biffi A, Hoffmann E, Panhuyzan-Goedkoop N, Hoogsteen J, Delise P, Hoff PI, Pelicccia A (2006) Recommandations for participation in leisure-time physical activity and competitive sports of patients with arrhythmias and potentially arrhythmogenic conditions. Part II: Ventricular arrhythmias, channelopathies and implantable defibrillators. Eur J Cardiovasc Prev Rehabil 13:676–686

Chapter 21
A 53-Year-Old Recreational Jogger with Atrial Fibrillation

Hein Heidbüchel

Family and Personal History

This is an amateur 43-year-old runner. He had been a long distance runner since adolescence, usually recreational but also competitive between age 16 and 23. He still continued jogging, 2 to 3 times per week, 7–10 km each session.

The patient had an uneventful previous medical history. He had developed palpitations 5 years before our initial evaluation. The athlete described this feeling as skipped beats, periodically frequent, which caused some subjective hindrance but no other associated specific cardiac symptoms.

Over the last 2 months, however, he developed episodes of longer lasting irregular palpitations. They occurred both at rest and during exercise, without a specific trigger being identifiable. These episodes lasted for 1 min to 2 h. When the arrhythmia was present, the patient noticed a clear decrease in exercise tolerance. Moreover, he reported one dizzy spell during exercise. His family history revealed no sudden unexpected death, nor family members with a similar problem.

Physical Examination

Physical examination was normal, with a blood pressure of 132/82 mmHg.

12-Lead ECG

Because of recurrent palpitations, an extended ECG was recorded during his first consultation. It revealed an episode of atrial fibrillation (AF) which terminated after four beats during the recording (Fig. 21.1). After only two sinus beats on the ECG,

H. Heidbüchel (✉)
Department of Cardiology – Electrophysiology, University Hospital Gasthuisberg, University of Leuven, Herestraat 49, B-3000 Leuven, Belgium Europe
e-mail: hein.heidbuchel@uz.kuleuven.ac.be

A. Pelliccia (ed.), *Sports Cardiology Casebook*,
DOI 10.1007/978-1-84882-042-5_21, © Springer-Verlag London Limited 2009

Fig. 21.1 The 12-lead ECG during initial visit, showing atrial fibrillation which terminated after four beats on the tracing. After only two sinus beats on the ECG, a new episode of AF started, presumably by atrial ectopic beats which initially were accompanied by aberrant conduction

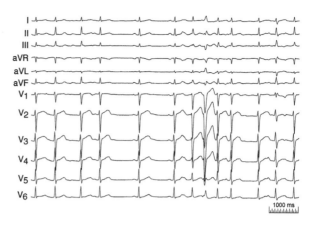

a new episode of AF started, presumably by atrial ectopic beats which initially were accompanied by aberrant conduction.

Echocardiography

Echocardiography showed normal cardiac dimensions and wall thickness. There was a trivial mitral regurgitation and a slightly enlarged left atrium (40 mm in the parasternal short axis view).

Diagnosis and Treatment

The AF was considered responsible for the symptoms of the patient and treatment was initiated with a low dose beta-blocker, i.e., metoprolol slow-release, 50 mg/day, to reduce the ventricular rate during AF episodes, in association with flecainide 2 × 100 mg/day for rhythm control.

Clinical Course

The athlete came to visit 1 month later. He had recurrent palpitations and mentioned one episode of exercise-induced pre-syncope (he did not feel palpitations at that moment). The ECG during that second visit is shown in Fig. 21.2. It showed a pattern of typical atrial flutter with predominant 2:1 atrio-ventricular conduction. After directed questioning, the athlete revealed that he had stopped beta-blocker therapy because of decreased exercise tolerance, but was still taking flecainide in monotherapy. Since there was suspicion for exercise-related arrhythmia episodes with high ventricular rate, a calcium channel blocker (verapamil 240 mg/day slow release) was added to the flecainide therapy.

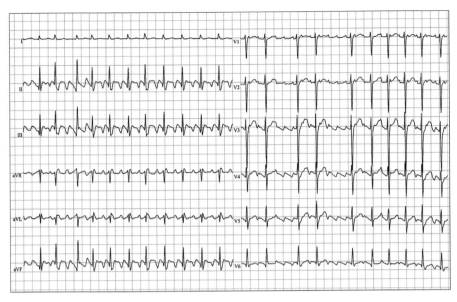

Fig. 21.2 One month after the first evaluation, the 12-lead ECG showed typical atrial flutter with predominant 2:1 atrio-ventricular conduction

Nevertheless, despite taking these drugs consistently, he collapsed at the end of a Sunday morning interval training in the woods. After recovery of consciousness he could crawl on hands and feet to his car and call emergency personnel with his mobile phone. They documented the ECG presented in Fig. 21.3, which showed a wide-QRS tachycardia at a rate of 250 bpm. After admission to the hospital the rhythm converted into atrial flutter with 2:1 conduction (with a similar atrial rate) before terminating spontaneously.

Discussion

This case illustrates how atrial fibrillation may organise into flutter, either intermittently and spontaneously or more easily under the influence of class 1 anti-arrhythmic drugs. In the latter case, it is referred to as "class-1 atrial flutter". Atrial flutter episodes may cause more hemodynamic compromise than atrial fibrillation, because of the risk for 1:1 AV conduction, particularly during exercise [1]. Although this can happen with all flutters, the situation is more common when flutter develops as a result of class 1 anti-arrhythmic drug treatment. In fact, class 1 drugs will slow the atrial rate of the flutter which facilitates 1:1 conduction, like in this case at the rate of 250 bpm (Fig. 21.3), whereas the original flutter had a rate of about 300 bpm in the atrium (Fig. 21.2). The rapid ventricular rate is associated with a very wide QRS due to profound intraventricular conduction delay as a result of the class 1 drug action, resembling VT from which it needs to be distinguished. The fast

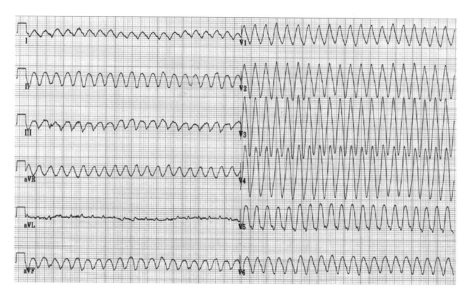

Fig. 21.3 The ECG on emergency admission a few weeks later, under treatment with flecainide 2 × 100 mg/day + verapamil slow-release 240 mg/day. The rhythm later converted to atrial flutter with 2:1 conduction (with a similar atrial rate) before terminating spontaneously

conducted flutter is associated with poor hemodynamic performance and can lead to cardiogenic shock and death.

Therefore, there is an absolute need to add AV nodal slowing drugs when treating atrial fibrillation in a recreational or competitive athlete. Of course, when atrial fibrillation occurs in an athlete, classical underlying causes have to be excluded, like thyroid dysfunction and, more frequently, systemic hypertension. If present, they should be treated appropriately. In general, approval for competitive sports participation in athletes with atrial fibrillation will depend on the tolerance of the arrhythmia during exercise, i.e. if hemodynamic symptoms due to fast uncontrolled rates can be excluded. Given the fact that it is even more difficult to control the ventricular rate during atrial flutter (in this case 1:1 conduction developed despite 240 mg verapamil per day), prophylactic flutter ablation should be considered in athletes with AF (like this athlete after his first visit) [2]. In case flutter is documented, ablation is even considered mandatory, both in competitive and recreational athletes [3].

In this patient the first ECG revealed clear signs of so-called "focally-induced atrial fibrillation", where atrial ectopic beats, usually originating in the pulmonary vein region, trigger episodes of atrial fibrillation [4]. These patients may be considered for pulmonary vein isolation for ablation of AF. Although theoretically athletes are good candidates (because of the younger age and absence of underlying heart disease), the results and long term outcome of ablation in this selected group are not well known. The potential benefits and risks of the procedure should be discussed with the patient. At moment, it is believed that freedom from atrial fibrillation can be expected in a 50% of persistent and 80% of paroxysmal cases of AF.

Effective ablation could allow termination of all anti-arrhythmic and bradycardia-inducing drugs and, therefore, complete resumption of competitive sports activity.

One has to consider, however, that an association has been described between endurance sports activity in adult and senior athletes (but not in the elite young competitors) [5] and development of atrial fibrillation [6]. The causes for this association are not known, but may reflect autonomic and/or structural atrial remodelling in adult and senior individuals associated with prolonged sports activity.

Therefore, it is unknown whether resumption of a full athletic activity after ablation could result in renewed/further risk for atrial remodelling and recurrence of atrial fibrillation in senior athletes. It has been shown that continuation of endurance sports may be an independent risk factor for development of atrial fibrillation after flutter ablation [7]. Therefore, it is sound to mention to the patient the opportunity to continue sport participation at decreased intensity and duration in order to potentially prevent further AF development.

References

1. Brembilla-Perrot B, Houriez P, Beurrier D, Claudon O, Terrier de la Chaise A, Louis P. Predictors of atrial flutter with 1:1 conduction in patients treated with class I antiarrhythmic drugs for atrial tachyarrhythmias. Int J Cardiol Aug 2001, 80(1):7–15
2. Nabar A, Rodriguez LM, Timmermans C, van den Dool A, Smeets JL, Wellens HJ. Effect of right atrial isthmus ablation on the occurrence of atrial fibrillation: observations in four patient groups having type I atrial flutter with or without associated atrial fibrillation. Circulation Mar 23 1999, 99(11):1441–1445
3. Heidbuchel H, Panhuyzen-Goedkoop N, Corrado D, Hoffmann E, Biffi A, Delise P, Blomstrom-Lundqvist C, Vanhees L, Ivarhoff P, Dorwarth U, Pelliccia A. Recommendations for participation in leisure-time physical activity and competitive sports in patients with arrhythmias and potentially arrhythmogenic conditions Part I: Supraventricular arrhythmias and pacemakers. Eur J Cardiovasc Prev Rehabil Aug 2006, 13(4):475–484
4. Haissaguerre M, Jais P, Shah DC, Takahashi A, Hocini M, Quiniou G, Garrigue S, Le Mouroux A, Le Metayer P, Clementy J. Spontaneous initiation of atrial fibrillation by ectopic beats originating in the pulmonary veins. N Engl J Med Sep 3 1998, 339(10):659–666
5. Pelliccia A, Maron BJ, Di Paolo FM, Biffi A, Quattrini FM, Pisicchio C, Roselli A, Caselli S, Culasso F. Prevalence and clinical significance of left atrial remodeling in competitive athletes. J Am Coll Cardiol 2005, 46:690–696
6. Mont L, Sambola A, Brugada J, Vacca M, Marrugat J, Elosua R, Pare C, Azqueta M, Sanz G. Long-lasting sport practice and lone atrial fibrillation. Eur Heart J Mar 2002, 23(6):477–482
7. Heidbuchel H, Anne W, Willems R, Adriaenssens B, Van de Werf F, Ector H. Endurance sports is a risk factor for atrial fibrillation after ablation for atrial flutter. Int J Cardiol Feb 8 2006, 107(1):67–72

Chapter 22
Paroxysmal Atrial Fibrillation in a Professional Cyclist

François Carré

Family and Personal History

This is a 33-year-old professional male cyclist. On February 15th, 2006 he underwent the annual medical and cardiovascular check-up in our Institute required for continuing professional cycling. Familial history revealed no known congenital or other cardiovascular diseases and no known cases of premature (<50 years) sudden cardiac death in close relatives. Personal history showed no exercise related cardiovascular symptoms, thoracic pain, dizziness, or palpitations. However, exercise bronchial hyper-responsiveness had been documented and treated with terbutaline and budesonide for 6 years.

Athletic History

The athlete started competitive cycling at the age of 17 years and had been engaged at professional level in the last 7 years. At the time of our evaluation, his training schedule included between 30,000 and 33,000 km per year, and this program had been in practice during the last 5 years. He was in good athletic condition and ready for the new athletic season.

Physical Examination

The physical examination showed normal findings on heart and lung auscultation. The resting heart rate was 40 bpm. The blood pressure was 120/70 mmHg. The height was 173 cm, the weight was 65 kg and the calculated fat mass was 10%.

F. Carré (✉)
Department of Physiology, Unité di Biologie et de Médecine du Sport, Pontchaillou Hospital*,*.
Rennes 1 University, INSERM U 642, France
e-mail: francois.carre@univ-rennes1.fr

A. Pelliccia (ed.), *Sports Cardiology Casebook*,
DOI 10.1007/978-1-84882-042-5_22, © Springer-Verlag London Limited 2009

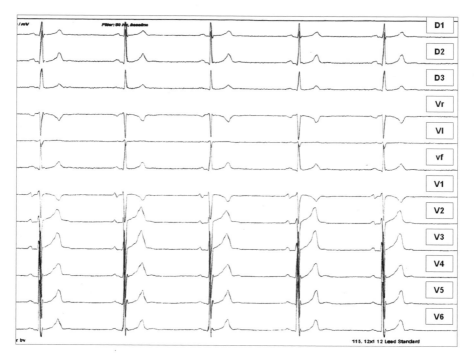

Fig. 22.1 Initial 12-lead resting ECG on February 2006

12-Lead ECG

Sinus bradycardia with 37 bpm was recorded, judged to be consistent with the high level of training. The PR, QRS, and QT/QTc intervals, respectively 175 ms, 104 ms and 429/363 ms were normal. T waves pattern were positive and tall in anterior precordial leads. A small intra-atrial conduction disturbance could be suspected because of slightly increased P wave duration (>100 ms), enlarged in lead II and a biphasic pattern in precordial lead V1 (Fig. 22.1).

Echocardiography

In accordance with the Union Cyclist International rule, a transthoracic echocardiography should performed every two years in this professional cyclist. The conclusion of echocardiographic study (Fig. 22.2) was consistent with athlete's heart diagnosis, showing a moderate and harmonious dilatation of the four cardiac chambers with normal resting systolic and diastolic function. Mild mitral and tricuspid insufficiencies were observed, without hemodynamic significance.

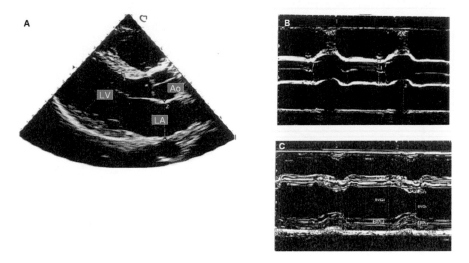

Fig. 22.2a–c Resting echocardiography. **a** 2D left-parasternal view of the left ventricle. **b** M-mode recording of the aorta and left atrium. **c** M-mode recording of left ventricle. LV = left ventricle; LA = Left atrium, Ao = aorta

Maximal Exercise Testing with Gas Analysis

A maximal exercise test with gas analysis was performed on an bicycle ergometer (Fig. 22.3). The maximal achieved workload was 410 W, with heart rate of 175 bpm, blood pressure 200/70 mmHg, maximal oxygen uptake 74.8 mL/min/kg, and oxygen pulse 28.8 mL O_2/beat.No symptoms, no arrhythmias and no repolarization abnormalities were observed. In conclusion, after the cardiovascular examination there was no reason for restricting the athlete from professional cycling.

Follow-Up and Other Testing

This cyclist had good sports results until June 2006. In June 2006 some brief exercise- induced palpitations were reported, which did not affect his physical performance. However, in August 2006 he was forced to withdraw from a cycling race because of palpitations, referred as a fast and irregular heart rate (180–210 bpm on personal heart rate monitor). For this reason, he went to the nearest hospital 24 h later. Clinical exam and 12-lead ECG showed a well tolerated atrial fibrillation (AF) with a ventricular rate between 90 and 110 bpm at rest (Fig. 22.4).

No prohibited drugs ingestion was admitted by the cyclist. Medical decision was to stop terbutaline and temporarily all sports practice. Blood testings (including thyroid parameters) were normal. The echocardiography was repeated but did no show changes compared to that performed in February.

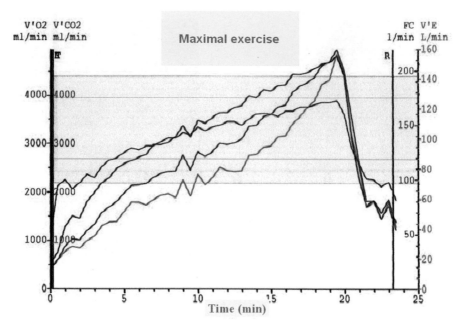

Fig. 22.3 Maximal exercise with expired gas analysis recorded on bicycle ergometer. $VO_2 = O_2$ uptake, $VCO_2 = CO_2$ production, Ve = ventilation; FC = heart rate

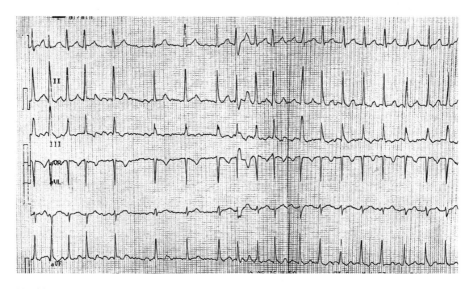

Fig. 22.4 12-lead ECG recorded during the paroxysmal atrial fibrillation on August 2006

Treatment and Recommendations

Acute treatment with oral amiodarone (two tablets twice daily) was instituted associated with nadroparine 0.6 mL/day. Sinus rhythm resumed within 12 h after the treatment. Re-evaluation could not reveal a primary underlying structural abnormality (no hypertension, heart disease, thyroid dysfunction). Medical treatment (acetylsalicylate and amiodarone) was progressively decreased and stopped one month later. At the same time, the athlete stopped sports practice for a three-months period.

During that period no events occurred and the cyclist started again with a moderate and progressively increasing physical training program.

Subsequent Follow-Up

Four months later, the athlete underwent the annual pre-season cardiovascular evaluation, which showed no abnormalities. No significant arrhythmia was noted during exercise test nor during 24 h Holter recording, which included a strenuous training session. The cyclist began a new race season in March 2007, but three other symptomatic paroxysmal (lasting less than 12 h) AF episodes occurred from July to September 2007.

At that time, we had a long dialogue with the cyclist. We explained the nature of the arrhythmia and commented that his athlete's heart and the high level of training might favor the emergence of paroxysmal AF. We gave him information about the possibility of pulmonary vein isolation or left atrial ablation in order to continue his professional career. However, he declined this proposal because he was concerned of the associated risks. On the other hand, chronic pharmacology treatment did not seem to us a good indication in this case for allowing competitive sport activity. We suggested the patient to continue sports practice at a lower level under appropriate drugs control. However, the cyclist preferred to stop his high level competitive sport, because of the incapacity to maintain a good level of performance without arrhythmias, the refusal to decrease his level of training, and his relatively old athletic age.

Discussion

This case illustrates the not uncommon occurrence of symptoms related to paroxysmal AF in a adult, highly trained athlete. In such circumstance, it is important to evaluate symptoms as the expression of AF, to exclude underlying causes, and to know the ventricular rate during AF. A temporary ineligibility is advisable during the time the athlete is being evaluated to exclude underlying cardiac diseases potentially responsible for the arrhythmia. In particular, an arrhythmogenic substrate should be investigated, such as Wolf-Parkinson-White syndrome, cardiomyopathies, myocarditis, unknown systemic hypertension, or use of prohibited drugs. Obviously, in case of structural cardiac disease the treatment and sports eligibility will be in accordance with that disease. In the most common instances, when AF is idiopathic and presents single or only rare episodes, and ventricular rate is not higher than maximal heart rate attained during exercise, the resumption of sport activity is possible without treatment [1]. Periodic (yearly) follow-up is advised. Instructions to stop physical activity if palpitations associated with symptoms of hemodynamic compromise (dizziness, unusual fatigue) arise must be given.

The patient should be informed about benefits and limitation of the procedure of pulmonary vein isolation and radiofrequency ablation. A more limited therapeutic option may be possible in selected cases, with ablation of the inferior isthmus in order to avoid the risk of atrial flutter arising during AF episode, especially in athletes that are treated with class-1 anti-arrhythmic drugs. In case of very fast ventricular rate and/or major symptoms, with athlete willing to resume competitive sport, radiofrequency ablation is advisable. After successful ablation, a short period of 1−3 months of observation, without symptoms and AF or flutter recurrence, is suggested before competitive sports be resumed. Indeed, a periodical (6 months) follow-up is recommended.

When the athlete with AF and very fast ventricular rate and/or major symptoms refuses the ablation procedure, or sport is reduced to leisure-time and non-competitive activity, treatment could be proposed with digoxin and calcium channels blockers, although these drugs are occasionally ineffective to maintain an appropriate heart rate. Beta-blockers are more efficient, but they have limitations in certain sports (altered performance and doping in some sports). Class 1 anti-arrhythmic drugs can be proposed with caution, as "pill in the pocket" therapeutic choice. In that instance, the athlete should refrain from intensive physical activity for two half-lives after ingestion, to avoid flutter with 1-to-1 A-V conduction [2].

Finally, anticoagulation depends on the classical risk factors for thromboembolic events. In case of anticoagulation treatment, sports with risk of body collision or trauma should be discouraged.

References

1. Pelliccia A, Fagard R, Bjørnstad HH, Anastassakis A, Arbustini E, Assanelli D, Biffi A, Borjesson M, Carrè F, Corrado D, Delise P, Dorwarth U, Hirth A, Heidbuchel H, Hoffmann E, Mellwig KP, Panhuyzen-Goedkoop N, Pisani A, Solberg E, van-Buuren F, Vanhees L. Rcommendations for competitive sports participation in athletes with cardiovascular disease. A consensus document from the Study Group of Sports Cardiology of the Working Group of Cardiac Rehabilitation and Exercise Physiology, and the Working Group of Myocardial and Pericardial Diseases of the European Society of Cardiology. Eur Heart J 2005, 26:1422−1445
2. Heidbuchel H, Panhuyzen-Goedkoop N, Corrado D, Hoffmann H, Biffi A, Delise P, Blomstrom-Lundqvist C, Vanhees L, Ivarhoff P, Dorwath U, Pelliccia A. Recommendations for participation in leisure-time physical activity and competitive sports in patients with arrhythmias and potentially arrhythmogenic conditions: Part I: Supraventricular arrhythmias and pacemakers. Eur J Prev Cardiovasc Rehabil 2006, 13:475−484

Chapter 23
A Female Soccer Player with Unusual Fatigability and Ventricular Arrhythmia

Erik Ekker Solberg, Terje Halvorsen, Knut-Haakon Stensaeth, and Finn Hegbom

Medical History

This is a female soccer player competing at national and international level. She is living as a single, in apparently healthy condition and without known clustering of cardiac diseases in her family. She did not use any drugs. She often suffered from banal upper respiratory infections and had exercise-induced asthma for a period during adolescence. Beside her career as a soccer player, she was working as a sales representative. Usually she trained between 7 and 12 times a week, depending on being in low- or high-season of sport events.

In January 2006, she suffered from upper respiratory infection. Eventually she showed symptoms of bronchitis. At this time of the year in Norway it is usually cold and wintry and in the middle of the flu season. Infection had several recurrences throughout the winter, and she did not recover completely. She went through four distinct infectious periods, lasting several weeks each time during the winter period. She continued, however, to train during these episodes although at a moderate level.

She was able to report scarce medical information regarding these flu episodes, including the negativity of serology tests (Ebstein Barr virus Ig G positive, Ig M negative, were judged as non-significant). Sero-reactive protein (CRP) and white blood cell counts were normal. During the summer 2006 she had a long period of bronchitis and at this stage she definitively experienced a decreased working capacity. In September she had fever for one week and suffered from sinusitis. She played a match a few days after the fever. She played badly, felt stressed and completely out of shape. She experienced palpitations for the first time. At the beginning of October she was admitted to hospital for acute chest pain occurring during a match. She experienced numbness in her left arm. The team doctor noted that her heart rhythm was irregular.

E.E. Solberg (✉)
Diakonhjemmet Hospital, Medical Department, 0319 Oslo, Norway
e-mail: erik.solberg@diakonsyk.no

A. Pelliccia (ed.), *Sports Cardiology Casebook*,
DOI 10.1007/978-1-84882-042-5_23, © Springer-Verlag London Limited 2009

Diagnostic Testing

At admission to hospital she complained about chest pain. The physical examination was unremarkable. The electrocardiogram (ECG) showed sinus rhythm with frequent premature ventricular beats (PVBs) with LBBB morphology and vertical axis (Fig. 23.1). Blood samples showed normal values, including infection parameters. Echocardiography was normal. At an exercise testing, she reached 170 W, with normal hemodynamic response. On initial work loads, frequent PVBs were observed, which disappeared with increasing work load. No ST-segment changes were observed during the exercise testing (Fig. 23.2). It was concluded that "the findings with normal echocardiography, normal exercise testing and blood samples excluded myocarditis with a high level of confidence". The decreasing frequency of the number of PVB during the work load was considered a positive sign. No training

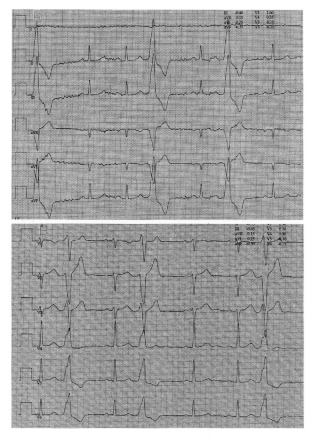

Fig. 23.1 Resting 12-lead ECG showing PVBs with left bundle branch configuration and inferior axis. The transition zone is between lead V_3 and V_4

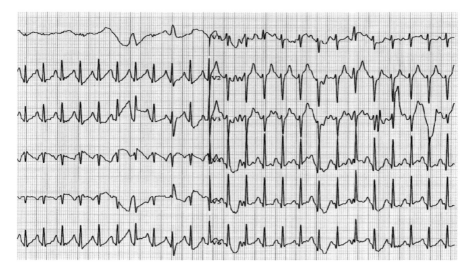

Fig. 23.2 Exercise ECG showing practically normal findings

restriction was advised to the patient, other than usual restriction during infection periods. No control was appointed.

Clinical Course

In November 2006, her clinical condition worsened. A Holter ECG monitoring was performed and showed sinus rhythm with frequent monomorphic PVBs, trigemini and bigemini, up to more than 34,000 PVBs/24 h. The PVBs morphology were unchanged (LBBB configuration and vertical axis). The transition zone was between lead V_3 and V_4. This suggested that arrhythmias had origin from a high site in the left ventricle outflow tract. About 1 month later, a new Holter ECG monitoring was recorded and the results were similar.

Recommendations and Treatment

She was advised to reduce substantially the training schedule, and restrict activity so as not to reach a pulse more than about 100 bpm. She was released on sick leave since she was unable to work because of tiredness and weakness. She also started treatment with beta blockers (Metoprolol 25 mg OD, increasing to 50 mg after a while), with a good symptomatic effect.

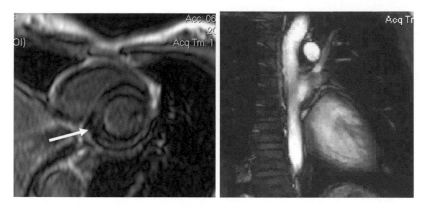

Fig. 23.3a,b Cardiac magnetic resonance showing gadolinium-late enhancement in the left myocardium (*arrow*)

Subsequent Clinical Course

After a few weeks she referred additional symptoms, including a near-syncope, feeling dizzy and dyspnoeic, and experienced diarrhoea. Echocardiography was repeated. The left ventricle was reported to be of normal size, without evidence of remodelling consistent with an athlete's heart. The ejection fraction was 52%. There was an insignificant tricuspid- and mitral regurgitation. Care was spent to assess the right ventricular morphology and function, and it was concluded that the right ventricle was normal in shape, structure and function.

In January 2007, cardiac magnetic resonance (CMR) was performed and no signs of ARVD were found. The CMR showed, however, a late enhancement (after i.v. gadolinium) centrally located in the left ventricle myocardium, a possible expression of an extensive inflammatory process. The ejection fraction was measured to be 49% (Fig. 23.3). Signal average ECG showed no presence of late potentials. At this stage the diagnosis of probable myocarditis primarily affecting the LV was made.

Recommendations and Treatment

Recommendation to avoid intense physical exercise and refrain from training was reiterated [1]. Drug treatment was also confirmed. A CMR-guided endomyocardial biopsy [2–4] was discussed. We considered that inflammation of the myocardium had lasted for at least 6 months and were afraid of a chronic course of the disease and possible evolution into a dilated cardiomyopathy [5, 6]. In the meanwhile, the athlete started to feel better and, despite medical advice, started to exercise again, with 30 min on a bike at slow speed and with light weights. She refrains at present from doing additional testing.

Discussion

This case offers a number of matters for consideration regarding the challenging diagnosis of myocarditis in a young athlete. Initially, suspicion for myocarditis arose clinically from the evidence of recurrent flu and careful research for myocardial lesion was performed. However, echocardiography failed to show morphologic or functional abnormalities, and blood tests were also negative. The exercise testing was performed without symptoms and only ventricular arrhythmia was present, which was misjudged not to be of clinical relevance because it disappeared during effort. When the clinical conditions of the athlete worsened, several clinical signs were present, including reduced capacity on exercise testing (that was much more remarkable in consideration of the previous superior capacity of the elite athlete), the reduced LV systolic function and a marked increase in frequency of ventricular arrhythmias. At that time, echocardiography was still unable to show significant morphologic alterations and only the CMR with late enhancement showed alterations that were considered suggestive for inflammation within the LV myocardium. Definitive evidence of myocarditis may be derived from histology and, for this reason, an indication to myocardial biopsy was discussed with a view to advise appropriate treatment [2–6]. However, in clinical practice, only a few athletes presenting with signs compatible with diagnosis of myocarditis (such as frequent ventricular arrhythmias and, even mild, LV dysfunction) eventually have a biopsy. So, in most instances, the challenging diagnosis of myocarditis remains the responsibility of the clinician, who also takes responsibility for consequent recommendations (withdrawal from sport and appropriate treatment).

References

1. Pelliccia A, Corrado D, Bjørnstad HH, Panhuyzen-Goedkoop N, Urhausen A, Carre F, Anastasakis A, Vanhees L, Arbustini E, Priori S. Recommendations for participation in competitive sport and leisure-time physical activity in individuals with cardiomyopathies, myocarditis and pericarditis.Eur J Cardiovasc Prev Rehabil Dec 2006, 13(6):876–885
2. Basso C, Carturan E, Corrado D, Thiene G. Myocarditis and dilated cardiomyopathy in athletes: diagnosis, management, and recommendations for sport activity. Cardiol Clin Aug 2007, 25(3):423–429
3. Chimenti C, Pieroni M, Frustaci A. Myocarditis: when to suspect and how to diagnose it in athletes. J Cardiovasc Med Apr 2006, 7(4):301–306 (Review)
4. Cooper LT, Baughman KL, Feldman AM, Frustaci A, Jessup M, Kuhl U, Levine GN, Narula J, Starling RC, Towbin J, Virmani R. American Heart Association; American College of Cardiology; European Society of Cardiology; Heart Failure Society of America; Heart Failure Association of the European Society of Cardiology. The role of endo-myocardial biopsy in the management of cardiovascular disease: a scientific statement from the American Heart Association, the American College of Cardiology, and the European Society of Cardiology. Endorsed by the Heart Failure Society of America and the Heart Failure Association of the European Society of Cardiology. J Am Coll Cardiol. Nov 6 2007, 50(19):1914–1931
5. Magnani JW, Dec GW. Myocarditis: current trends in diagnosis and treatment. Circulation Feb 14 2006, 113(6):876–890 (Review)
6. Narula N, McNamara DM. Endo-myocardial biopsy and natural history of myocarditis. Heart Fail Clin Oct 2005, 1(3):391–406 (Review)

Chapter 24
A 38-Year-Old Marathon Runner with Tricuspid Valve Regurgitation

A.W. Treusch, O. Oldenburg, T. Butz, A. Fründ, E. Oepangat, F. van Buuren, and K.-P. Mellwig

Personal Medical History

This is a 38-year-old male marathon runner who presented in November 2006 in our Heart Department for second opinion regarding the presence of tricuspid valvular regurgitation and implications for participation in marathon racing. The patient reported no discomfort and trained regularly and without limitations. He reported a previous diagnosis of valve disease in 2001 in a routine check-up by the local cardiologist. Besides deep venous thrombosis after long flight in January 2005, there were no relevant issues. He takes no medication, no drugs, or nicotine.

Family History

Mother and father suffer from systemic hypertension. There is no family history of myocardial infarction, coronary artery disease, stroke, heart failure or sudden cardiac death.

Type and Level of Sports Activity Performed

He is an ambitious leisure time marathon runner. The usual training schedule included 10 km distance runs, two to three times per week with a controlled heart rate of 150–160 bpm. Best marathon running time is 4 h 20 min. He had no relevant sport associated injuries.

A.W. Treusch (✉)
Department of Cardiology, Leopoldina Hospital, Gustav-Adolf-Str. 8, D – 97422 Schweinfurt, Germany
e-mail: atreush@hdz.nrw.de

A. Pelliccia (ed.), *Sports Cardiology Casebook*,
DOI 10.1007/978-1-84882-042-5_24, © Springer-Verlag London Limited 2009

Physical Examination

The patient was a 38-year-old white male in no apparent distress. He was alert and oriented to all qualities. Normal body-structure 174 cm, 89 kg. Heart was regular in rate and rhythm with 56 bpm. The blood pressure was 102/90 mmHg. There were normal heart sounds. A 2/6 systolic murmur was present on apex and Erb with augmentation on deep inspiration. No diastolic murmur was fund. Pulses on both sides were equivalent. No relevant findings on head, neck and throat. The lungs were clear on auscultation. The palpation of the abdomen revealed no relevant findings. No lymph nodes or suspect areas visible or palpable.

Patient referred a previous diagnosis of "valve disease" not better specified and, based on physical examination, suspicion raised for tricuspid valve regurgitation.

Diagnostic Testing

12-Lead ECG

Regular sinus rhythm with 56 bpm, QRS main-vector 82°, pattern of incomplete right bundle branch block, with QRS widening to 110 ms. No evidence for left or right ventricular hypertrophy (Fig. 24.1a,b).

Echocardiography

Normal left ventricular (LV) dimensions without regional wall thickening. Normal LV cavity shape and dimensions. Normal systolic function, in the absence of wall motion anomalies. Moderately dilated left atrium. Right ventricle and right atrium showed moderate enlargement. Tricuspid valve (TV) appeared to be morphologically normal, but moderate TV regurgitation was seen. Calculated pul-

a   **b**

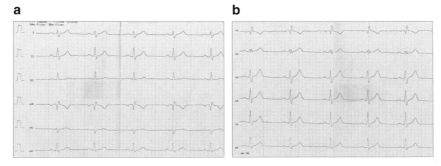

Fig. 24.1a,b 12-lead ECG shows sinus rhythm with 56 bpm, QRS main-vector 82°, pattern of incomplete right bundle branch block, with QRS widening to 110 ms. No evidence for *left* or *right* ventricular hypertrophy

monary pressure was at upper normal limits (PAP peak 32 mmHg) (Fig. 24.2). All other valves were normal in morphology and function. There was a enhanced motion of the interatrial septum, without Doppler signs of a shunt (Video 24.1).

Video 24.1a,b Two-dimensional and Doppler echocardiography (4-chamber apical view). Tricuspid valve (TV) appeared to be morphologically normal, but moderate TV regurgitation was seen. There was a enhanced motion of the interatrial septum, without Doppler signs of a shunt

Fig. 24.2 CW Doppler echocardiography recorded from the 3rd intercostal space of left sternal border. The peak CW flow exceeds 3 m/s and calculated pulmonary artery pressure (PAP peak 32 mmHg) was at upper normal limits

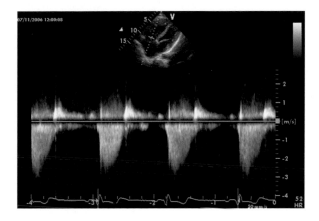

Treadmill – Exercise – Testing

Test performed on a treadmill starting at 8 km/h with increments of 2 km/h per 3 min. Exhaustion after 12 min at 14 km/h. Heart rate at rest 89 bpm, at peak exercise 193 bpm. Blood pressure at rest 120/90 mmHg, at peak exercise 180/60 mmHg. Blood pressure and heart rate behaviour during exercise were normal. No pathologic ECG changes during exercise were found. Oxygen consumption (VO_2) at anaerobic threshold was 42.1 mL/kg/min. Peak-VO_2 was 48.6 mL/kg/min representing 135% of the predicted VO_2-max. Lactate at rest 1.1 mmol/L, at peak 13.9 mmol/L.

In conclusion: no cardio respiratory limitation and excellent physical performance (Fig. 24.3).

Cardiac Magnetic Resonance (CMR)

The LV dimensions and function were normal. Borderline left atrial dimensions. There is mild right atrial and right ventricular enlargement. Moderate tricuspid valve regurgitation was evident. No right-to-left- or left-to-right-shunts were fund at level of atrial septum. No abnormal pulmonary veins, no sinus-venous-defect or coronary-sinus-defect (Video 24.2).

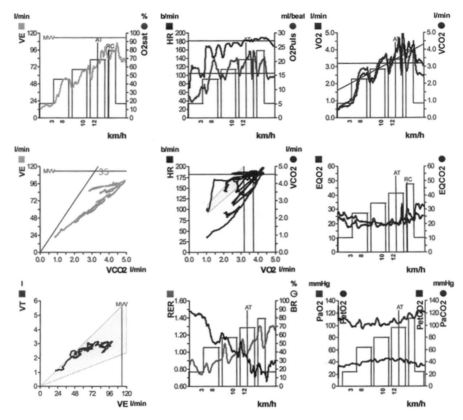

Fig. 24.3 Cardiopulmonary testing. Oxygen consumption (VO$_2$) at anaerobic threshold was 42.1 mL/kg/min. Peak-VO$_2$ was 48.6 mL/kg/min representing 135% of the predicted VO$_2$-max. Lactate at rest 1.1 mmol/L, at peak 13.9 mmol/L

Video 24.2 Cardiac magnetic resonance. Cardiac dimensions were as follows. Left ventricle: EDD 55 mm, ESD 35 mm, EDV 138 mL, EDVi 68 mL/m^2, ESV 45 mL, ESVi 22 mL/m^2, SV 93 mL, EF 67%. Right ventricle: EDD 42 mm, ESD 38 mm, EDV 271 mL, EDVi 133 mL/m^2, ESV 109 mL, ESVi 53 mL/m^2, SV 162 mL, EF 60%

ECG Holter Monitoring

Sinus rhythm over the 24-h recording. Minimum heart rate of 42 bpm and a maximum heart rate of 189 bpm (during exercise). During night time sinus pauses were observed up to 2.7 s during intermittent second degree, type 1 AV-Block. No other rhythm disturbances were seen (namely, atrial fibrillation or tachyarrhythmias).

Laboratory Results

Normal values for electrolytes, liver, renal, CRP, cholesterols, BNP, urine analysis, White blood count, Haemoglobin, platelets, coagulation, iron, thyroid and HbA1, HbA1c.

Diagnosis and Recommendations

Final diagnosis was idiopathic, moderate tricuspid valve regurgitation with no signs of right ventricular dysfunction or pulmonary hypertension. This condition was considered compatible with the athlete lifestyle and, specifically, did not represent, *per se*, sufficient reason for stopping running training and competition. However, continued clinical surveillance was needed and periodical follow-up was requested.

Discussion

According to the results of diagnostic testing, the case presented here had a moderate regurgitation of the tricuspid valve, on a morphologically normal valve, without significant increase in pulmonary pressure, which does not require medical or surgical treatment. Discussion was focused on the potential impact of the continued sport activity on the natural course of this abnormality, i.e., the potential worsening of the valve lesion due to hemodynamic overload associated with long-distance running. In the absence of definite information on this field, we carefully considered the pros and cons of our decision; in particular, we believed unlikely that long-distance running up to 10 km in an amateur athlete may cause substantial worsening of the valve dysfunction; therefore, the patient was informed that sport activity can be continued. However, we also believed prudent to follow periodically the patient and required a close monitoring (every 6 months). The patient was fully informed of the considerations surrounding his case and, finally, endocarditis prophylaxis was recommended according to standard protocol [1].

Reference

1. Pelliccia A, Fagard R, Bjørnstad HH, Anastassakis A, Arbustini E, Assanelli D, Biffi A, Borjesson M, Carrè F, Corrado D, Delise P, Dorwarth U, Hirth A, Heidbuchel H, Hoffmann E, Mellwig KP, Panhuyzen-Goedkoop N, Pisani A, Solberg E, van-Buuren F, Vanhees L. Recommendations for competitive sports participation in athletes with cardiovascular disease. A consensus document from the Study Group of Sports Cardiology of the Working Group of Cardiac Rehabilitation and Exercise Physiology, and the Working Group of Myocardial and Pericardial Diseases of the European Society of Cardiology. Eur Heart J 2005, 26:1422–1445

Chapter 25
A Young Rower with an Unusual Left Ventricular Hypertrophy

Filippo M. Quattrini, Fernando Maria Di Paolo, Cataldo Pisicchio, Roberto Ciardo, and Antonio Pelliccia

Family and Personal History

This 18-year-old male, elite rower was referred for cardiologic evaluation to our Institution for the presence of abnormal repolarization pattern on the 12-lead ECG, performed elsewhere in the setting of national preparticipation screening program. The athlete was engaged in daily training sessions of approximately 6 hours(h), mostly on the water but also in the gym. He had competed in several international events, including Olympic Games, and was gold and silver medallist in the World Rowing Championship. The personal history was negative for symptoms or cardiac disease. The father had systemic hypertension with mild renal dysfunction. No other known cardiovascular diseases or premature (<50 years) sudden cardiac death among relatives were reported.

Physical Examination

On physical examination weight was 92 kg, height 1.82 m and blood pressure was 120/70 mmHg. No heart murmurs or abnormal sounds were present at cardiac auscultation.

12-Lead ECG

The 12-lead ECG showed sinus rhythm. Marked repolarization abnormalities with T wave inversion in anterior precordial leads, from V1 to V4, and flattened T wave in V5 were present. In addition, minor right ventricular conduction delay was observed (Fig. 25.1).

F.M. Quattrini (✉)
Institute of Sport Medicine and Science, Italian National Olympic Committee, Department of Sport Medicine, Largo Piero Gabrielli, 1 00197, Rome, Italy
e-mail: f.quattrini@guest.coni.it

A. Pelliccia (ed.), *Sports Cardiology Casebook*,
DOI 10.1007/978-1-84882-042-5_25, © Springer-Verlag London Limited 2009

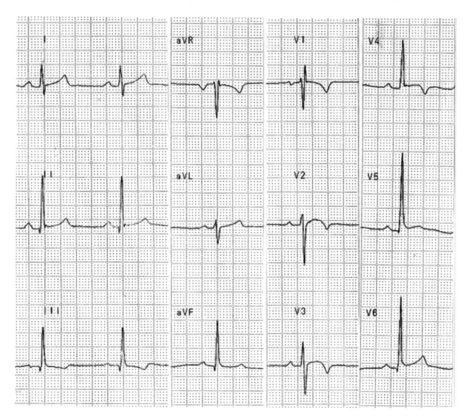

Fig. 25.1 12-lead rest ECG recorded in the athlete during training period. Repolarization abnormalities are present in anterior precordial leads (V1 to V4)

Echocardiography

Echocardiography showed mild Left Ventricular (LV) hypertrophy, homogenously distributed, with maximum LV wall thickness of 13 mm on anterior and posterior ventricular septum. LV end-diastolic cavity dimension was 50 mm. Systolic function was normal (EF 65%) in the absence of wall motion abnormalities. No alteration of filling pattern was observed with trans-mitral Doppler echocardiography (Fig. 25.2). No abnormalities in right ventricular morphology or wall motion suggestive for arrhythmogenic right ventricular cardiomyopathy were observed.

Exercise Testing

On exercise testing performed with cycloergometer, starting from 40 W with increments of 40 W every 2 min, the athlete reached 280 W, with maximum heart rate 170 bpm and with normal behavior of blood pressure (at peak exercise:

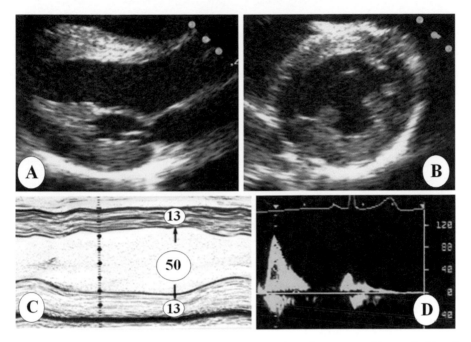

Fig. 25.2 **a,b** Two-dimensional echocardiographic view from the parasternal long axis (**a**) and short axis (**b**) of left ventricle. **c** M-mode dimensions of the ventricular septum, posterior free wall, and end-diastolic cavity size of left ventricle. **d** The trans-mitral Doppler flow

200/80 mmHg). No arrhythmias were observed during exertion. The repolarization pattern with T-wave inversion in precordial leads remained unchanged during exertion, without ST-segment changes and no symptoms suggestive for inducible ischemia.

In consideration of the presence of abnormal ECG pattern and LV hypertrophy, with the aim to exclude the presence of hypertrophic cardiomyopathy (HCM) and achieve evidence that morphological LV characteristics were compatible with "athlete's heart", we required the athlete to stop training and competition for a short period.

Detraining

After 3 months of complete detraining the athlete was re-evaluated in our Institution. The 12-lead ECG, although not completely normal, showed reduction of repolarization abnormalities previously observed in precordial leads V4–V5 (Fig. 25.3). Echocardiography showed partial regression of LV hypertrophy (maximum LV wall thickness decreased from 13 to 11 mm) and a trivial increment of LV end diastolic dimension (from 50 to 52 mm; Fig. 25.4). Based on these findings, we believed that LV hypertrophy observed in this case was a consequence of a physiologic cardiac

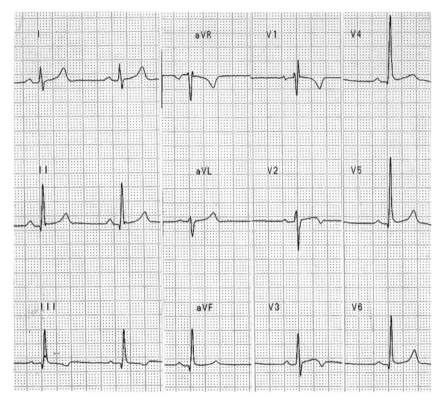

Fig. 25.3 12-lead resting ECG recorded in the same athlete after 3 months of detraining. Repolarization abnormalities in anterior precordial leads (V1 to V4) are partially regressed

adaptation to intensive training, and the athlete was allowed to resumed full competitive sport.

Clinical Course

Over the subsequent 8 years of follow-up, during which serial cardiologic evaluations were performed, including repeated 12-lead ECGs and echocardiograms, no significant changes in the ECG pattern or changes in LV dimensions were observed, and athlete remained asymptomatic. After 8 years of continued athletic career, at age of 27 years, the athlete referred *de novo* occurrence of palpitations during exercise.

Additional Diagnostic Testing

A new cardiologic evaluation was therefore performed, including exercise testing and echocardiography. During exercise testing, the athlete developed the

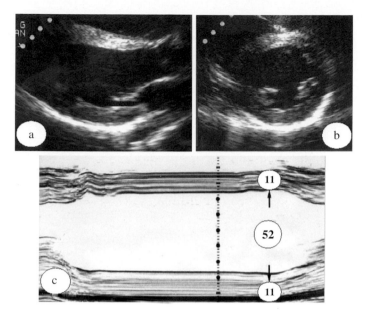

Fig. 25.4a–c Two-dimensional echocardiographic views and M-mode dimensions from the same athlete after 3 months of detraining. **a** Parasternal long axis view. **b** Parasternal short axis view. **c** M-mode derived LV dimensions

same symptoms as recently experienced, which corresponded to a short, fast run (190 bpm) of wide QRS tachycardia on the electrocardiogram (Fig. 25.5). Echocardiography confirmed the presence of mild LV hypertrophy (maximum LV wall thickness 13 mm), as previously observed, normal LV cavity size and, for the first time, a mild systolic anterior motion (SAM) of mitral valve (Video 25.1).

Video 25.1 Two-dimensional echocardiographic long-axis and short-axis views of the same athlete at the most recent evaluation showing mild SAM (A) and mild, diffuse LV hypertrophy (maximum LV wall thickness 13–14 mm)

Additional testing was performed, including exercise nuclear scintigraphy, which showed normal myocardial perfusion and normal LV systolic function at rest and during exercise. The ventriculo coronaro-angiography did not show any significant lesion of coronary vessels, but a short and non-occluding myocardial bridge on distal portion of left anterior descending coronary artery was evident (Fig. 25.6).

Diagnosis and Recommendations

The presence of abnormal repolarization pattern on 12-lead ECG, LV hypertrophy with initial SAM of the mitral valve, in association with myocardial bridge and exercise-induced tachyarrhythmia were judged consistent with a probable diagnosis

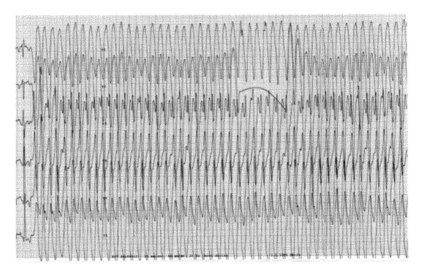

Fig. 25.5 Electrocardiogram recorded during exercise testing, showing a short burst of fast wide QRS tachycardia

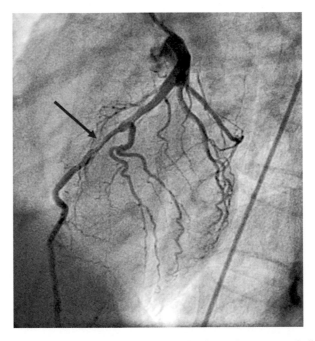

Fig. 25.6 Coronaro-angiography of the same athlete, showing a short, non occluding myocardial bridge on distal portion of left anterior descending coronary artery (*arrow*)

of HCM. Therefore, the athlete was disqualified from competitive sport according to the Italian and European recommendations, closely resembling those reported by the Bethesda Conference #36 [1, 2].

Discussion

This case illustrates one of the most compelling issue that arises in sports cardiologist practice: i.e., the differential diagnosis between physiological LV hypertrophy and mild phenotypic expressions of HCM. The diagnosis of HCM was controversial in this case, in consideration that a mild LV hypertrophy was expected to be present in a highly trained athlete and the repolarization changes in the 12-lead ECG are not an uncommon finding in elite athletes [3]. However, certain characteristics of this case were not consistent with diagnosis of athlete's heart and should have raised suspicion for a non-physiologic LV hypertrophy. On initial evaluation, LV cavity dimension was within normal limits (and not enlarged, as expected in a highly trained rower) in spite of a substantial thickening of LV wall and, moreover, LV cavity size did not reduce after detraining. In this case, our diagnosis of physiologic LV hypertrophy was mostly based on the reduction of LV wall thickness after detraining [4]. Indeed, none of the common alterations of HCM were present at that time, such as left atrial enlargement, alteration of diastolic filling pattern, or systolic anterior motion of mitral valve [5, 6].

With regard to ECG changes, this finding was not unexpected. In a previous study of a large cohort of elite athletes, Pelliccia reported prevalence of abnormal ECG patterns in 60%, including 14% with distinctly abnormal ECGs [7]. In a more recent study, the same author [8] reported that athletes showing distinctly abnormal patterns, such as that described in our case, may develop morphologic evidence of cardiomyopathics (mostly HCM) during a long period of follow-up. Therefore, it may be that morphologic cardiac changes suggestive for HCM may require a long-term follow-up before being clearly evident [8]. Another point to be considered was the localization of ECG repolarization abnormalities in anterior precordial leads, from V1 to V4, which suggested right ventricular abnormalities (absent at imaging testing).

The diagnosis of probable HCM in this athlete was based on the presence of mild LV hypertrophy, systolic motion of mitral valve and myocardial bridging. Myocardial bridging occurs in patients with HCM, with a prevalence as high as 30% [9]. In young HCM patients, presence of myocardial bridging is associated with chest pain, cardiac arrest and ventricular tachycardia. No association is reported between presence and length of myocardial bridging and the extent of LV hypertrophy [10, 11].

Finally, our decision for disqualification was also based on the recognition that sport activity may itself represent a risk for acute cardiac events (including sudden death). This could be promoted by specific variables related to stress of sports, e.g., electrolyte imbalance, hemodynamic and autonomic changes, as well as other still undefined mechanisms. Therefore, a competitive athlete with HCM judged to be "low risk" in the absence of traditional risk markers, may nevertheless be at unacceptably increased risk solely by virtue of involvement in high intensity competitive sports, as shown by the tragic case of the soccer player Marc Vivien Foé [12].

References

1. Pelliccia A, Fagard R, Bjørnstad HH, Anastassakis A, Arbustini E, Assanelli D, Biffi A, Borjesson M, Carrè F, Corrado D, Delise P, Dorwarth U, Hirth A, Heidbuchel H, Hoffmann E, Mellwig KP, Panhuyzen-Goedkoop N, Pisani A, Solberg E, van-Buuren F, Vanhees L. Recommendations for competitive sports participation in athletes with cardiovascular disease. A consensus document from the Study Group of Sports Cardiology of the Working Group of Cardiac Rehabilitation and Exercise Physiology, and the Working Group of Myocardial and Pericardial Diseases of the European Society of Cardiology. Eur Heart J 2005, 26:1422–1445
2. Maron BJ, Zipes DP. 36th Bethesda Conference: Eligibility recommendations for competitive athletes with cardiovascular abnormalities. J Am Coll Cardiol 2005, 45:2–64
3. Maron BJ, Pelliccia A. The heart of trained athletes: cardiac remodelling and the risks of sports, including sudden death. Circulation 2006, 114:1633–1644
4. Pelliccia A, Maron BJ, De Luca R, et al. Remodelling of left ventricular hypertrophy in elite athletes after long-term deconditioning. Circulation 2002, 105:944–949
5. Klues HG, Schiffers A, Maron BJ. Phenotypic spectrum and patterns of left ventricular hypertrophy in hypertrophic cardiomyopathy: morphologic observations and significance as assessed by two-dimensional echocardiography in 600 patients. J Am Coll Cardiol 1995, 26:1699–1708
6. Maron BJ. Hypertrophic cardiomyopathy: a systematic review. JAMA 2002, 287:1308–1320
7. Pelliccia A, Maron BJ, Culasso F, Di Paolo FM, Caselli G, Biffi A, Piovano P. Clinical significance of abnormal electrocardiographic patterns in trained athletes. Circulation 2000, 102:278–284
8. Pelliccia A, Di Paolo FM, Quattrini FM, et al. Outcomes in athletes with marked ECG repolarization abnormalities. N Engl J Med 2008, 358:152–161
9. Alegria JR, Herrmann J, Holmes DR Jr, et al. Myocardial bridging. Eur Heart J 2005, 26:1159–1168
10. Yetman AT, McCrindle BW, MacDonald C, et al. Myocardial bridging in children with hypertrophic cardiomyopathy – a risk factor for sudden death. N Engl J Med 1998, 339:1201–1209
11. Feld H, Guadanino V, Hollander G, et al. Exercise-induced ventricular tachycardia in association with a myocardial bridge. Chest 1991, 99:1295–1296
12. Maron BJ. Sudden death in young athletes. N Engl J Med 2003, 349:1064–1075

Chapter 26
An Elite Athlete with Controversial Left Ventricular Hypertrophy

Barbara Di Giacinto, Fernando Maria Di Paolo, and Antonio Pelliccia

Medical History

This 17-year-old male athlete underwent cardiovascular evaluation in our Institute for the first time in 1995, selected as member of the national swimming team, based on his excellent athletic results. In the personal history no cardiac symptoms or previous cardiovascular diseases were reported. The family history was negative for known cardiovascular diseases and sudden cardiac death in close relatives.

Physical Examination

On physical examination there was a healthy male, height 182 cm, weight 78 kg, blood pressure 120/80 mmHg. Cardiac sounds were normal; a mild systolic murmur over the left ventricular (LV) outflow tract was noted.

12-Lead ECG

The ECG showed normal sinus rhythm with 58 bpm; PR interval was 0.16 s and corrected QT interval was 0.42 s. No significant morphologic abnormalities were noted, with possible exception of mildly inverted T wave in aVL, and biphasic in peripheral lead I and in V2 and small Q wave in standard leads III and aVF (Fig. 26.1).

Echocardiography

On echocardiogram LV cavity was within normal limits (end-diastolic diameter = 50 mm) with normal shape, maximum walls thickness 11−12 mm in the anterior

B. Di Giacinto (✉)
Institute of Sport Medicine and Science, Italian National Olympic Committee, Department of Sport Medicine, Largo Piero Gabrielli, 1 00197 Rome, Italy
e-mail: barbara.digiacinto@virgilio.it

A. Pelliccia (ed.), *Sports Cardiology Casebook*,
DOI 10.1007/978-1-84882-042-5_26, © Springer-Verlag London Limited 2009

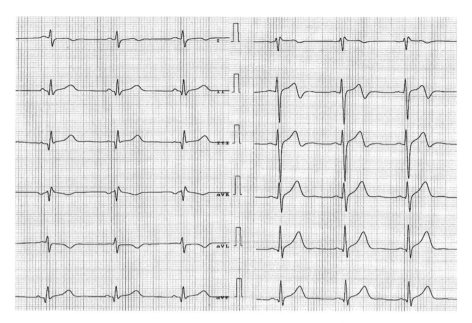

Fig. 26.1 12-lead ECG of the athlete recorded at initial evaluation (1995): normal sinus rhythm is present with 58 bpm; PR interval is 0.16 s and corrected QT interval is 0.42 s. Mildly inverted T wave in aVL, in V2 and small q wave in standard leads III and aVF are evident

ventricular septum (Fig. 26.2). LV systolic function was normal (EF = 62%), in the absence of wall motion abnormalities. Normal LV filling pattern was seen at Doppler echocardiography. No anomalies were observed in the right ventricle. The overall picture was considered consistent with athlete's heart and the athlete was cleared for competitive sport participation.

Clinical Course

In the following years, the athlete continued his career as an elite competitor by participating at World Championships and Olympic Games, with outstanding achievements. At the same time, usually before participation in these events, he underwent periodical cardiovascular evaluations in our Institute. No changes were noted in the 12-lead ECG pattern and echocardiographic findings and no cardiovascular symptoms or events in the family members occurred until 2001 (7 years after the initial evaluation, at age of 24). At that time, the athlete reported rare and occasional feeling of irregular heart beats.

The ECG Holter monitoring was then performed and 175 premature ventricular beats (PVBs) with two morphologies were recorded in 24 h. The exercise testing showed a few, isolated PVBs, in the absence of other ECG abnormalities. Echocardiography demonstrated a thickened ventricular septum (maximum wall thickness

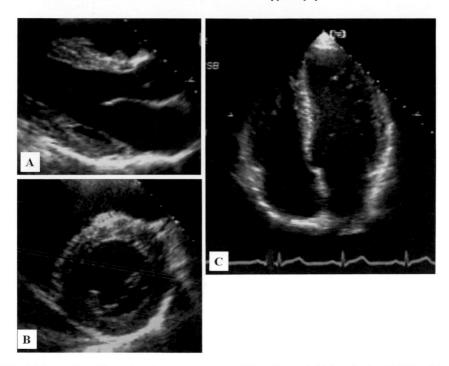

Fig. 26.2a–c Two-dimensional echocardiogram of the athlete at initial evaluation (1995). **a** The parasternal long axis view. **b** Parasternal short axis view. **c** The four chamber view. LV cavity shows a normal size (end-diastolic diameter = 50 mm), with normal shape and mildly increased walls thickness (maximum wall thickness = 11–12 mm in the anterior ventricular septum)

= 13 mm), with normal cavity size and shape. LV systolic function was normal (ejection fraction 70%) and diastolic filling pattern was normal. The overall pattern was still considered consistent with physiologic cardiac remodeling induced by intensive athletic conditioning. However, a close follow-up (every 6 months) was required.

In the subsequent 1-year period the athlete underwent serial evaluations, including repeated 24-h ECG Holter monitoring and echocardiograms. One of these Holter monitoring showed a short episode of NSVT (Fig. 26.3), one couplet of PVBs and two isolated PVBs. No changes were seen in the resting 12-lead ECG or in cardiac morphology as assessed by echocardiography.

The arrhythmia was not considered, *per se*, sufficient reason for disqualification and the athlete continued his successful career with periodical controls. Several ECG Holter monitoring performed over 2 subsequent years showed rare PVBs.

On October 2003, at age of 26, the athlete underwent a cardiovascular control before his participation in the 2004 Olympic Games. At that time, the 12-lead ECG pattern was unchanged. However, certain alterations were observed at echocardiography: LV cavity appeared relatively smaller than previously observed (end-diastolic diameter = 48 mm), associated with more substantial wall thickening,

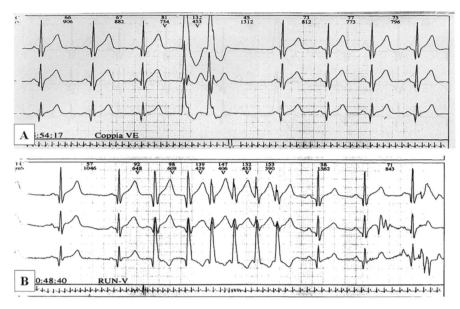

Fig. 26.3a,b 24-h ECG Holter monitoring recorded during the follow-up. **a** One couplet of PVBs is shown. **b** A short episode of NSVT (6 beats; minimum RR interval 390 ms)

which appeared to affect disproportionately the ventricular septum and anterior free wall (maximum wall thickness = 14 mm). LV systolic function and diastolic filling pattern were still normal (Fig. 26.4, Videos 26.1, 26.2, and 26.3).

The morphologic features raised suspicion for a non-physiologic LV hypertrophy, and diagnosis of hypertrophic cardiomyopathy (HCM) was debated. The athlete was informed of the clinical suspicion and potential implication regarding his athletic career and he decided to have a different opinion by several consultant cardiologists. In the course of the cardiologist consultations, new diagnostic testing were performed.

Cardiac magnetic resonance showed a more substantial hypertrophy than seen with echocardiography, i.e., the anterior free wall and anterior ventricular septum were disproportionately thickened (18−24 mm) in comparison to posterior and inferior free wall (11−14 mm). Indeed, delayed hyper-enhancement with postgadolinium was seen within the hypertrophic septum, suggesting presence of intramyocardial fibrosis.

Myocardial biopsy was done in four specimens. Myocardial disarray with myocytes architecture displaced by increased interstitial fibrosis and hypertrophic myocytes were seen. Large perivascular fibrosis and spotted focal areas of fibrous replacement were present. Some of the arterioles showed a moderate thickening of the media layer. The overall histologic pattern was consistent with diagnosis of HCM.

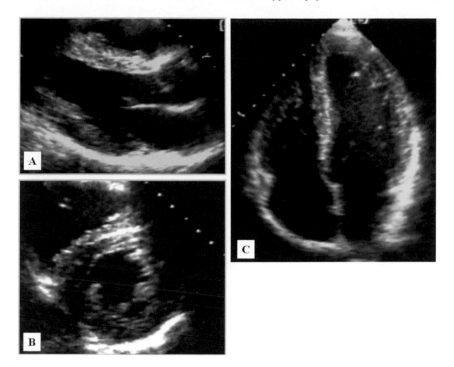

Fig. 26.4a–c Two-dimensional echocardiogram of the same athlete at most recent evaluation (2003). **a** The parasternal long axis view. **b** Parasternal short axis view. **c** The four chamber view. LV cavity appears relatively smaller than previously measured (end-diastolic diameter = 48 mm), associated with more substantial wall thickening, which appeared to affect disproportionately the ventricular septum and anterior free wall (maximum wall thickness = 14 mm)

Videos 26.1–3 Comparative echocardiographic views of the same athlete recorded in 1995 and 2003. In the 1995 study, LV cavity is of normal size (end-diastolic diameter = 50 mm) with normal walls thickness (11–12 mm) and normal function

Genetic study: DNA analysis of MYBPC3 gene was performed to assess the presence of gene abnormalities potentially responsible for HCM. A mutation in myosin binding protein C was found, with change GAA>CAA in esone 17 (E542Q).

Family screening: both parents and brother underwent cardiac screening for HCM. The brother, 30 years old, and the father, 52 years old, showed normal 12-lead ECG and echocardiography. The mother, aged 50, showed a normal 12-lead ECG; on echocardiography LV cavity size was normal, but wall thickness was 11–12 mm in the posterior ventricular septum, and prominent papillary muscles and enlarged left atrium (transverse diameter, 43 mm) were observed. These phenotypic findings were judged compatible, although not diagnostic, with mild phenotypic expression of HCM.

Diagnosis and Recommendations

The final diagnosis was HCM and, based on the widely accepted recommendations for athletes with CV disease [1, 2], the athlete was disqualified from competitive sport participation. Consequently, he retired from training and competitions and spend his athletic experience in the training and management of young athletes. No symptoms or events had occurred after cessation of the athletic career during the subsequent 4-year period.

Discussion

This case shows how difficult can be the differential diagnosis between athlete's heart and HCM in an individual athlete, in particular when the phenotypic expression of HCM is characterized by only mild LV hypertrophy. The suspicion of HCM in this athlete did not arise at first evaluation, despite mild changes noted on the 12-lead ECG and echocardiography. Specifically, the 12-lead ECG showed the selective presence of inverted T wave in aVL, which is not common pattern in trained athletes. No concern arose either from the presence of a mild q wave in inferior standard leads. These mild changes were considered at that time as consistent with the athlete's heart.

In young patients with HCM, however, ECG abnormalities may for a long time precede the phenotypic appearance of the disease [3, 4]. Recent data from our group showed that athletes with abnormal repolarization pattern, in the absence of morphologic evidence for cardiac disease, may develop over time morphologic and clinical evidence of arrhythmogenic cardiomyopathies responsible for adverse events (such as cardiac arrest) [5]. Therefore, an abnormal ECG pattern in an athlete with borderline LV hypertrophy mandates serial clinical and imaging controls. The echocardiographic features of this athlete (normal LV cavity with mild LV wall thickening) were interpreted for long time as consequence of the athletic conditioning and did not raise clinical concern [6, 7]. However, the morphologic LV pattern observed in this athlete was somehow different from that usually observed in other elite swimmers. In the patient's teammates, the LV cavity dimension was usually more enlarged (i.e., end-diastolic dimension >54 mm), in the presence of similar LV wall thickening (maximum 11 or 12 mm).

The premonitory marker for the underlying structural cardiac disease was the presence of rare but complex ventricular arrhythmia, which occurred several years before the appearance of morphologic cardiac changes. Diagnosis became evident in the follow-up only with different diagnostic testing, namely cardiac magnetic resonance. By this technique, a more substantial LV wall thickening than observed by echocardiography was seen, with prominent LV hypertrophy in the anterior free wall, area which was poorly visualized by echocardiography. This observation supports the added value of cardiac magnetic resonance when the interpretation of LV hypertrophy is controversial. Indeed, the evidence of late hyper-enhancement together with the presence of myocardial fibrosis was further support for HCM diagnosis [8].

The finding of gene abnormality made unequivocal the interpretation of previous diagnostic testing. However, gene analysis was performed late in the diagnostic course, when diagnosis of HCM was already done based on imaging technique and histology assessment. The gene analysis was positive for myosin binding protein C mutation, which anomaly is not uncommonly found in patients with late development of LV hypertrophy in adult age [9, 10], such as was the case with this athlete, who showed wall thickening increasingly late in adult age.

Another consideration which is related to this case is the potential role of a continued athletic career in triggering (or enhancing) the phenotypic expression of the underlying gene abnormality: although there is no proof, we cannot exclude that continued participation in training and competition might have an impact in promoting LV wall thickening. Late development of LV hypertrophy in athletes suggests continued clinical surveillance (with imaging testing) in young individuals with borderline, controversial LV hypertrophy.

When diagnosis of HCM was unequivocal, the decision to disqualify the athlete from competition was controversial on clinical ground. In fact, the athlete was asymptomatic, the family history was negative for sudden death, the LV hypertrophy was only mild, the arrhythmia was rare and the hemodynamic response to exercise testing was excellent. According to the usual criteria for risk stratification in HCM, this athlete should have considered at "low risk". The question arose therefore whether we had the right to interrupt his superb athletic career (with loss of all benefits, including economic revenues) just before the Olympics.

We based our decision on the current recommendations, i.e., the Italian Guidelines, the ESC and BC #36 Recommendations [1, 2], which state that athletes with HCM should be excluded from most competitive sports (with the possible exception of those characterized by low static, low dynamic intensity, such as golf). These recommendations are based on the assumption that competitive sports participation may *itself* constitute a risk factor for sudden death in HCM, usually due to ventricular tachyarrhythmias in susceptible young individuals [11]. Sudden death could be promoted by specific variables related to stress of sports, e.g., electrolyte imbalance, hemodynamic and autonomic changes, as well as other still undefined mechanisms. A competitive athlete with HCM judged to be "low risk" in the absence of traditional risk markers may nevertheless be at unacceptably risk solely by virtue of involvement in high intensity competitive sports, as was shown by the sudden death of the professional soccer player Marc Vivien Foè from Cameroon [12].

References

1. Pelliccia A, Fagard R, Bjornstad HH, Anastassakis A, Arbustini E, Assanelli D, Biffi A, Borjesson M, Carre F, Corrado D, Delise P, Dorwarth U, Hirth A, Heidbuchel H, Hoffmann E, Melwig KP, Panhuyzen-Goedkoop NM, Pisani A, Solberg EE, Vanbuuuren F, Vanhees L. Recommendations for competitive sports participation in athletes with cardiovascular disease. Eur Heart J 2005, 26:1422–1445

2. Maron BJ, Zipes Douglas P. 36th Bethesda Conference: Eligibility Recommendations for Competitive Athletes with Cardiovascular Abnormalities. JACC 2005, 45(8):1318–1321.
3. Panza JA, Maron BJ. Relation of electrocardiographic abnormalities to evolving left ventricular hypertrophy in hypertrophic cardiomyopathy during childhood. Am J Cardiol 1989, 63:1258–1265
4. Montgomery JV, Harris KM, Casey SA, Zenovich AG, Maron BJ. Relation of electrocardiographic patterns to phenotypic expression and clinical outcome in hypertrophic cardiomyopathy. Am J Cardiol 2005, 96:270–275
5. Pelliccia A, Di Paolo FM, Quattrini FM, et al. Outcomes in athletes with marked ECG repolarization abnormalities. N Engl J Med Jan 10 2008, 358(2):152–161
6. Pelliccia A, Maron A, Maron J, et al. The upper limits of physiological cardiac hypertrophy in highly trained elite athletes. N Engl J Med Jan 31 1991, 324(5):295–301
7. Maron BJ, Pelliccia A. The heart of trained athletes: cardiac remodeling and the risks of sports including sudden death. Circulation 2006, 114:1633–1644
8. Rickers C, Wilke NM, Jerosch-Herold M, et al. Utility of cardiac magnetic resonance imaging in the diagnosis of hypertrophic cardiomyopathy. Circulation 2005, 112:855–861
9. Maron BJ, Niimura H, Casey SA, Soper MK, Wright GB, Seidman JG, Seidman CE. Development of left ventricular hypertrophy in adults with hypertrophic cardiomyopathy caused by cardiac myosin-binding protein C gene mutations. J Am Coll Cardiol 2001, 38:315–321
10. Richard P, Charron P, Carrier L, et al. Hypertrophic cardiomyopathy: distribution of disease genes, spectrum of mutations, and implications for a molecular diagnosis strategy. Circulation 2003, 107(17):2171–2174
11. Corrado D, Basso C, Rizzoli G, Schiavon M, Thiene G. Does sport activity enhance the risk of sudden death in adolescents and young adults? J Am Coll Cardiol 2003, 42:1959–1963
12. British Broadcasting Cooperation. Midfielder Marc-Vivien Foe dies after collapsing during an international in France. news.bbc.co.uk/sport1/hi/football/3024360.stm

Chapter 27
A Non-compaction Cardiomyopathy or Innocent LV Trabeculation?

Cataldo Pisicchio, Filippo M. Quattrini, Fernando Maria Di Paolo, Roberto Ciardo, and Antonio Pelliccia

Medical History

This is a 17-year-old male, elite tennis player. The athlete has been playing at national level since the age of 12, participating in several national and international events. For his results, he was selected for inclusion in the Italian national team. Therefore, he underwent medical evaluation in our Institute, in accord to the mandate of the Italian National Olympic Committee. The athlete had been previously evaluated and cleared at national pre-participation screening program. His training program included daily training sessions of approximately 7 hours (h).

Family and Personal History

The personal history was negative for cardiovascular diseases and symptoms. The mother had systemic hypertension. No other cardiovascular diseases or known cases of premature (<50 years) sudden cardiac death among close relatives were reported.

Physical Examination

On physical examination his weight was 71 kg, height 1.76 m and blood pressure 125/80 mmHg. No murmurs or abnormal heart sounds were present at cardiac auscultation.

C. Pisicchio (✉)
Institute of Sport Medicine and Science, Italian National Olympic Committee, Department of Sport Medicine, Largo Piero Gabrielli, 1 00197 Rome, Italy
email: aldopis@gmail.com

A. Pelliccia (ed.), *Sports Cardiology Casebook*,
DOI 10.1007/978-1-84882-042-5_27, © Springer-Verlag London Limited 2009

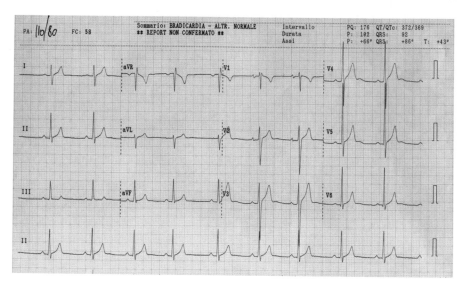

Fig. 27.1 12-lead ECG showing sinus rhythm of 58 bpm and normal morphology; i.e., absence of conduction delays, atrial enlargement or repolarization abnormalities

12-Lead ECG

12-lead ECG showed sinus rhythm with a mean heart rate 55 bpm. Normal cardiac electric axis, normal AV conduction (PQ 0.17 s) and normal QTc interval (0.38 s) were observed. No repolarization abnormalities were evident (Fig. 27.1).

Exercise Testing

On exercise testing performed with bicycle-ergometer, starting from 40 W with increments of 40 W every 2 min, the athlete reached 240 W, with maximum heart rate 174 bpm and normal blood pressure (at peak: 200/80 mmHg) (Fig. 27.2). Only two premature ventricular beats (PVBs), with a left bundle branch block and superior axis morphology were observed during the recovery period. Normal ST-segment pattern and T-wave were observed, and no symptoms were induced by exercise. In order to exclude the presence of more serious ventricular arrhythmia occurring during the specific athletic activity, we decided to obtain a 24-h ECG monitoring.

24-h ECG Holter Monitoring

Only two supraventricular premature beats (SVPBs) and no ventricular arrhythmias were present at 24-h Holter monitoring, including a specific tennis session lasting for about 2 h.

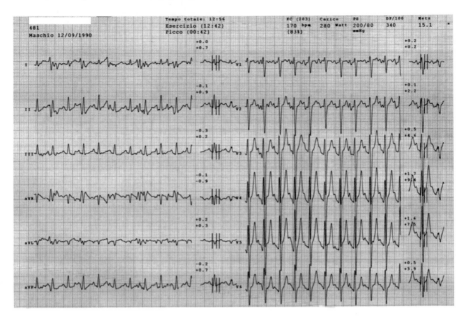

Fig. 27.2 12-lead ECG at peak of exercise. The ST-T pattern is normal and no arrhythmias were found

Signal Averaging ECG

The exam was negative for the presence of ventricular late potentials (Fig. 27.3).

Echocardiography

Echocardiographic findings showed normal left ventricular (LV) end-diastolic cavity size (55 mm) with wall thickness within normal limits (anterior and posterior ventricular septum 11 mm and posterior free wall 10 mm). Global systolic function was normal (EF 62%) in the absence of wall motion abnormalities. Normal filling pattern was detected by trans-mitral Doppler echocardiography. Within LV cavity, at mid-apical level of anterior, lateral, posterior and inferior walls, multiple trabeculations, deep intertrabecular recesses communicating with the ventricular cavity were observed. Prominent trabecular network was seen in the right ventricle, too. (Fig. 27.4; Video 27.1 a,b).

Video 27.1 a,b Two-dimensional short axis echocardiographic view of left ventricle at level of middle-apical region. A large area of pseudo-hypertrophy is evident, with recesses and trabeculations. **c,d** Subcostal and four-chamber apical echocardiographic views

Video 27.2 a,b The CMR (short axis view **(a)** and horizontal long-axis view **(b)**) confirms the evident trabecular pattern within the left and right ventricular cavities, without evidence of myocardial recesses or isolated thinning of the myocardial walls

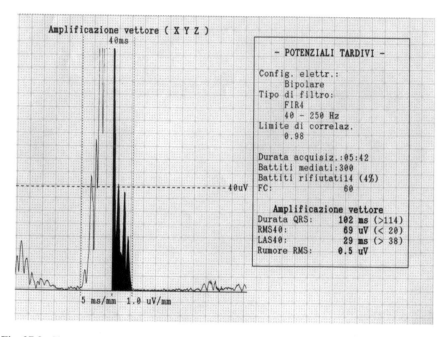

Fig. 27.3 Signal averaging ECG showing absence of late potentials

Cardiac Magnetic Resonance (CMR)

This testing confirmed the evidence of prominent trabecular meshwork at level of middle and apical region, without images suggestive for non-compaction myocardium. The right ventricle presented prominent trabecular network, too. No evidence of signal intensity alteration within LV myocardium were observed. The LV showed normal absolute cavity dimensions with wall-thickness at upper normal limits. No global systolic dysfunction or segmental wall motion abnormalities were found (Fig. 27.5; Video 27.2 a,b).

Diagnosis and Recommendations

Based on the results of CMR the diagnosis of LV noncompaction was unlikely and we defined this morphologic pattern as prominent trabeculations in the absence of familial and clinical evidence of the disease. In consideration of the absence of symptoms and family occurrence of cardiomyopathies, the normal 12-lead ECG

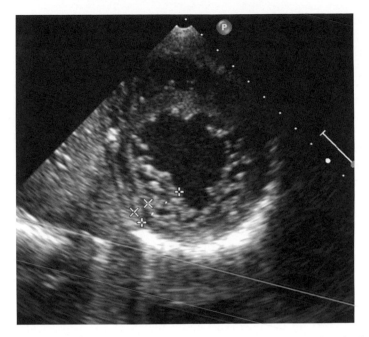

Fig. 27.4 Two-dimensional short axis echocardiographic view of left ventricle at level of apical region, just below the papillary muscles. A large area of pseudo-hypertrophy is evident at level of lateral and inferior wall, with recesses and trabeculations

Fig. 27.5 Cardiac magnetic resonance. In the distal region of both the left and right ventricular cavities, a large trabecular pattern is evident. The prominent trabecular patterns expands towards the cavity, but no thinning of the free ventricular walls are evident

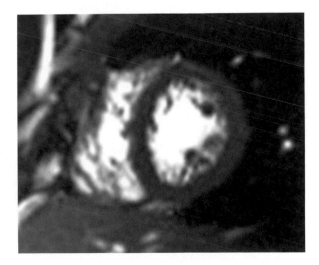

pattern, absence of arrhythmias and excellent cardiovascular adaptation to effort, we believed that there were no reason to disqualify the athlete from competition and, therefore, we cleared him with the recommendation to have serial, periodical controls.

Discussion

LV non-compaction (LVNC) is considered as unclassified cardiomyopathy [1–3], characterized by spongy myocardium, consequence of incomplete myocardial morphogenesis, with persistence of trabeculations and deep recesses. On the basis of echocardiographic studies, its prevalence has been estimated to be 0.05% in the general population [4]. Familial cases account for up to 50% of cases in various published series, and the inheritance mechanism is autosomal dominant in majority of such cases. X linked or mitochondrial transmission was also found [5–7]. Diagnosis of non-compaction myocardium can be made by echocardiography. Criteria for diagnosis are the presence of multiple trabeculations, with deep recesses communicating with the ventricular cavity [8–12] and an increased ratio between non-compacted to compacted wall in systole (>2.0 in adults and >1.4 in children.). In our case, suggestive echocardiographic images for non-compaction myocardium were present. The present case underlines the challenge of differential diagnosis in borderline cases, where morphologic appearances are at border of criteria to identify non-compaction myocardium and differentiate from trabeculations, which can represent an innocent variant of normal LV morphology.

In our case, we relied most on CMR imaging, which showed a prominent trabecular meshwork in the middle to apical region of LV, without clear images of thinning LV wall and non-compaction myocardium. The CMR is supposed to have superior imaging quality than echocardiography [13–15], and the ratio of non-compacted to compacted myocardium (NC/C ratio) of >2.3 in diastole has been proposed as threshold for diagnosis of pathological non-compaction (with values for specificity and negative predictions of 99%) [16]. In our athlete, despite the echocardiographic images suggestive for LV noncompaction, no other typical structural cardiac abnormalities were present [17–19], and the ECG pattern was normal, without changes commonly associated with non-compaction (T wave inversions, WPW pattern, arrhythmias, or conduction abnormalities) [20, 21]. Finally, no clinical manifestations commonly reported in LVNC, such as heart failure, ventricular tachycardia, cardio-embolic events, or syncope were present in our case [22–25]. At present, no definite recommendations are available for these patterns, at the border between pathologic LV non-compaction and prominent but innocent LV trabeculation. Therefore, caution in applying the present example to clinical practice is needed, and efforts should be made by the examining physician to tailor precise advice to a single athlete-patient. In the future, additional information may also derive from DNA testing: search of the genes G4.5, FKB12 and Alpha-Dystrobrevin seems to be associated with LV noncompaction [26–28].

References

1. Agmon Y, Connolly HM, Olson LJ, Khandheria BK, Seward JB. Noncompaction of the ventricular myocardium. J Am Soc Echocardiogr 1999, 12(10):859–863
2. Cavusoglu Y, Ata N, Timuralp B, Gorenek B, Goktekin O, Kudaiberdieva G, et al. Noncompaction of the ventricular myocardium: report of two cases with bicuspid aortic valve

demonstrating poor prognosis and with prominent right ventricular involvement. Echocardiography 2003, 20(4):379–383

3. Chin TK, Perloff JK, Williams RG, Jue K, Mohrmann R. Isolated noncompaction of left ventricular myocardium. A study of eight cases. Circulation 1990, 82(2):507–513

4. Ritter M, Oechslin E, Sutsch G, Attenhofer C, Schneider J, Jenni R. Isolated noncompaction of the myocardium in adults. Mayo Clin Proc 1997, 72:26–31

5. Digilio MC, Marino B, Bevilacqua M, Musolino AM, Giannotti A, Dallapiccola B. Genetic heterogeneity of isolated noncompaction of the left ventricular myocardium. Am J Med Genet 1999, 85(1):90–91

6. Johnson MT, Zhang S, Gilkeson R, Ameduri R, Siwik E, Patel CR, et al. Intrafamilial variability of noncompaction of the ventricular myocardium. Am Heart J 2006, 151(5):1012 e7–14

7. Bleyl SB, Mumford BR, Brown-Harrison MC, Pagotto LT, Carey JC, Pysher TJ, et al. Xq28-linked noncompaction of the left ventricular myocardium: prenatal diagnosis and pathologic analysis of affected individuals. Am J Med Genet 1997, 72(3):257–265

8. Bodiwala K, Miller AP, Nanda NC, Patel V, Vengala S, Mehmood F, et al. Live three-dimensional transthoracic echocardiographic assessment of ventricular noncompaction. Echocardiography 2005, 22(7):611–620

9. Borregnero LJ, Corti R, de Soria RF, Osende JI, Fuster V, Badimon JJ. Images in cardiovascular medicine. Diagnosis of isolated noncompaction of the myocardium by magnetic resonance imaging. Circulation 2002, 105(21):E177–178

10. Canale J, Cortes Lawrenz J, Moreno Valenzuela FG. Spongy cardiomyopathy in an elderly woman. Echocardiographic description. Arch Cardiol Mex 2005, 75(2):184–187

11. Cavusoglu Y, Tunerir B, Birdane A, Timuralp B, Ata N, Gorenek B, et al. Transesophageal echocardiographic diagnosis of ventricular noncompaction associated with an atrial septal aneurysm in a patient with dilated cardiomyopathy of unknown etiology. Can J Cardiol 2005, 21(8):705–707

12. Daimon Y, Watanabe S, Takeda S, Hijikata Y, Komuro I. Two-layered appearance of noncompaction of the ventricular myocardium on magnetic resonance imaging. Circ J 2002, 66(6):619–621

13. Biagini E, Ragni L, Ferlito M, Pasquale F, Lofiego C, Leone O, et al. Different types of cardiomyopathy associated with isolated ventricular noncompaction. Am J Cardiol 2006, 98(6):821–824

14. Finsterer J, Stolberger C, Kopsa W. Noncompaction in myotonic dystrophy type 1 on cardiac MRI. Cardiology 2005, 103(3):167–168

15. Finsterer J, Stollberger C. Cardiac MRI versus echocardiography in assessing noncompaction in children without neuromuscular disease. Pediatr Radiol 2006, 36(7):720–721; author reply 722–723

16. Robson JMF, Anderson RH, Watkins H, Neubauer S, Petersen SE, Selvanayagam JB, Wiesmann F, Matthew D. Left ventricular non-compaction: insights from cardiovascular magnetic resonance imaging. J Am Coll Cardiol 2005, 46:101–105

17. Ilercil A, Barack J, Malone MA, Barold SS, Herweg B. Association of noncompaction of left ventricular myocardium with Ebstein's anomaly. Echocardiography 2006, 23(5):432–433

18. Gambetta K, Cui W, El-Zein C, Roberson DA. Anomalous left coronary artery from the right sinus of valsalva and noncompaction of the left ventricle. Pediatr Cardiol 2008, 29(2): 434–437

19. Friedman MA, Wiseman S, Haramati L, Gordon GM, Spevack DM. Noncompaction of the left ventricle in a patient with dextroversion. Eur J Echocardiogr 2007, 8(1):70–73

20. Salerno JC, Chun TU, Rutledge JC. Sinus bradycardia, Wolff Parkinson White, and left ventricular noncompaction: an embryologic connection? Pediatr Cardiol 2008, 29(3): 679–682

21. Kawasaki T, Azuma A, Taniguchi T, Asada S, Kamitani T, Kawasaki S, et al. Heart rate variability in adult patients with isolated left ventricular noncompaction. Int J Cardiol 2005, 99(1):147–150

22. Yan CW, Zhao SH, Lu MJ, Jiang SL, Wei YQ, Li SG, et al. Clinical characterizations of patients with isolated left ventricular noncompaction diagnosed by magnetic resonance imaging. Zhonghua Xin Xue Guan Bing Za Zhi 2006, 34(12):1081–1084

23. Fazio G, Corrado G, Pizzuto C, Zachara E, Rapezzi C, Sulafa AK, et al. Supraventricular arrhythmias in noncompaction of left ventricle: is this a frequent complication? Int J Cardiol 2008, 127(2): 255–256

24. Alehan D. Clinical features of isolated left ventricular noncompaction in children. Int J Cardiol 2004, 97(2):233–237

25. Fichet J, Legras A, Bernard A, Babuty D. Aborted sudden cardiac death revealing isolated noncompaction of the left ventricle in a patient with Wolff-Parkinson-White syndrome. Pacing Clin Electrophysiol 2007, 30(3):444–447

26. Finsterer J, Stollberger C. Genetic heterogeneity of noncompaction. Chin Med J 2007, 120(18):1647; author reply 1648

27. Nakamura T, Colbert M, Krenz M, Molkentin JD, Hahn HS, Dorn GW II, et al. Mediating ERK 1/2 signaling rescues congenital heart defects in a mouse model of Noonan syndrome. J Clin Invest 2007, 117(8):2123–2132

28. Corrado G, Checcarelli N, Santarone M, Stollberger C, Finsterer J. Left ventricular hypertrabeculation/noncompaction with PMP22 duplication-based Charcot-Marie-Tooth disease type 1A. Cardiology 2006, 105(3):142–145

Chapter 28
A 31-Year-Old Male, Recreational Soccer Player with "Low Risk" Hypertrophic Cardiomyopathy

Pietro Delise

Medical History

This is a 31-year-old male, amateur soccer player. The family history was positive for hypertrophic cardiomyopathy (HCM), which was initially identified in the grand father and subsequently in the father. His grandfather died at 52 years of age from cardiac failure. His father is still alive, 65 years old, with a well tolerated permanent atrial fibrillation. The patient medical history started with a syncope at age of 6, when for the first time he underwent a comprehensive cardiovascular evaluation, which showed presence of obstructive HCM. Then, at age of 9, he underwent miotomy-miectomy for removal of the obstruction localized at basal portion of the ventricular septum. Subsequently, he had remained asymptomatic and without limitation in his usual day-to-day life, including participation in recreational soccer games. For that reason, at the age of 29 years he underwent a medical control.

Physical Examination

The physical evaluation was unremarkable. No murmurs or abnormal sounds were found. Brachial arterial pressure was 130/80 mmHg.

12-Lead ECG

The 12-lead ECG showed normal sinus rhythm. The ECG pattern was suggestive for left atrial enlargement and increased R/S wave voltages in precordial leads V2−V5 compatible with LV hypertrophy (Fig. 28.1).

P. Delise (✉)
Department of Cardiology, Ospedale di Conegliano, Hospital of Santa Maria dei Battuti, Via Flisati 66, 30171 Mestre (Venezia) Conegliano, Italy
e-mail: pietro.delise@libero.it

A. Pelliccia (ed.), *Sports Cardiology Casebook*,
DOI 10.1007/978-1-84882-042-5_28, © Springer-Verlag London Limited 2009

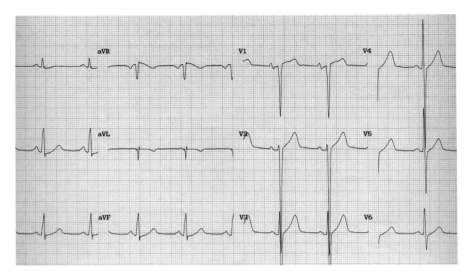

Fig. 28.1 12-lead ECG shows normal sinus rhythm. The ECG pattern shows P wave changes suggestive for left atrial enlargement and increased R/S wave voltages in precordial leads compatible with LV hypertrophy

Echocardiography

The LV diastolic cavity dimension was 46 mm, ventricular septum 19 mm, posterior free wall 9 mm, left atrium diameter 45 mm. Systolic function was within normal limits (EF = 55%). The study of diastolic function at transmitral Doppler flow and Tissue Doppler Imaging showed mild impairment of LV filling and relaxation.

Exercise Testing

The test was performed on the bicycle ergometer and the subject was able to achieve a peak workload of 200 W, with maximum heart rate 165 bpm, brachial arterial pressure 205/80 mmHg, in the complete absence of symptoms, ECG abnormalities of repolarization pattern, or arrhythmias.

ECG Holter Monitoring

The 24-h ECG Holter monitoring showed mean heart rate 64 bpm, 23 supraventricular premature beats, 357 ventricular premature beats and 3 ventricular couplets (shortest RR interval 400 ms).

Diagnosis and Recommendations

Diagnosis of HCM was confirmed on the basis of familial evidence and histology at the time of myotomy-myectomy. The patient was considered to be at low risk, based on the absence of symptoms and arrhythmias, normal blood pressure behaviour during exercise, mild LV hypertrophy and good physical performance. Therefore, he was reassured regarding the clinical course of the disease. Indeed, according to the ESC and Italian guidelines (which closely resemble the BC#36) competitive sport participation was denied [1, 2], but recreational sport activities (including soccer) was permitted.

Clinical Course

About 18 months after the medical evaluation the patient had a syncope while playing soccer. Emergency team was promptly requested and reached the place in about 5 min. A 12-lead ECG was recorded which showed ventricular fibrillation. Resuscitation manoeuvres were immediately started and defibrillation initiated. Over 15 shocks were delivered with only transient sinus rhythm resumption and rapid degeneration into ventricular fibrillation. Finally a stable sinus rhythm was obtained with ST segment elevation in anterior leads (Fig. 28.2), but the patient went into electromechanical dissociation and died.

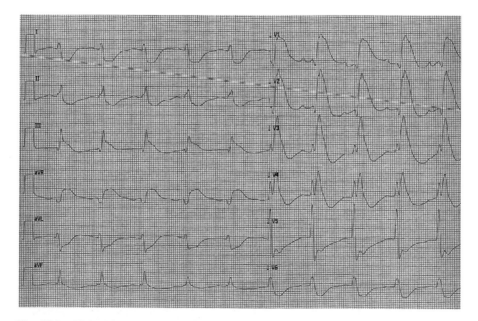

Fig. 28.2   12-lead ECG recorded during the resuscitation manoeuvre, after DC shock, shows sinus rhythm with prominent ST-segment elevation in anterior precordial leads and corresponding ST-segment depression in the lateral, inferior standard leads

Fig. 28.3 Autopsy specimen shows increased ventricular septum thickness (maximum thickness = 25 mm). Multiple small areas of fibrosis are evident in the postero-septal region of the ventricular septum

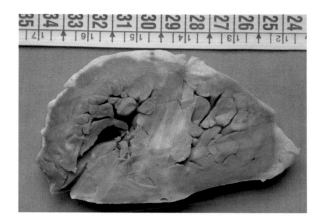

Autopsy Findings

The heart weight was 850 g. Maximum thickness measured at ventricular septum was 25 mm (Fig. 28.3). Multiple small areas of fibrosis were seen in the postero-septal region of the left ventricle, and were confluent into a large central area. On histology, diffuse contraction bands were detected. Coronary arteries were of normal size and free of significant atherosclerotic lesions.

Discussion

This patient was affected by familial HCM. The first manifestation of the disease occurred during childhood, with symptoms related to LV obstruction, which eventually justified surgery treatment. After septal myotomy-myectomy, he conducted a fairly normal life; namely, he had no symptoms and he was even able to participate in leisure time sport activities without limitations. At the time of our evaluation the athlete showed only mild LV hypertrophy, no evidence of LVOT obstruction and no significant arrhythmias either at rest or during maximal effort. Furthermore, he tolerated a high work load (i.e., 200 W) during exercise testing. The overall clinical picture was therefore consistent with a "low risk" HCM and persuaded his physician to allow participation in amateur sport activities, including soccer. Sudden death, however, occurred unexpectedly during effort due to ventricular fibrillation and, despite sinus rhythm restoration by prompt defibrillation, electro-mechanical dissociation ended in cardiac arrest. The autopsy demonstrated areas of post-necrotic fibrosis (in the presence of normal coronary arteries) and confirmed that silent small infarcts and recurrent episodes of ischemia had occurred during life. The ischemia-related fibrosis likely represented the morphologic substrate for occurrence of re-entry malignant tachyarrhythmia.

In conclusion, certain comments are relevant to this case, and are common to most young HCM patients:

1. The occurrence of sudden death in an HCM patient is unpredictable.
2. The absence of arrhythmias induced by laboratory testing (i.e., ECG Holter monitoring, exercise testing) does not reliably predict (or exclude) future occurrence of malignant ventricular arrhythmias.
3. The absence of symptoms (either at rest and during effort) does not warrant a low risk for cardiac arrest.
4. In young HCM patients engaged in sport activity the risk of sudden death cannot be assessed uniquely on commonly used clinical criteria. Sport activity represents, *per se*, a powerful risk factor in HCM patients, and can trigger sudden death by some exercise-related mechanisms (i.e., alteration in blood volume, hydration and electrolytes, as well as autonomic nervous changes) [3−5]. Therefore, competitive sport activity (with possible exception of certain low intensity activities) should be denied in young patients with HCM.
5. When cardiac arrest occurs in HCM patients, resuscitation is difficult and only occasionally successful, even in young patients without evidence of coronary flow impairment.

References

1. Pelliccia A, Fagard R, Bjørnstad HH, Anastassakis A, Arbustini E, Assanelli D, Biffi A, Borjesson M, Carrè F, Corrado D, Delise P, Dorwarth U, Hirth A, Heidbuchel H, Hoffmann E, Mellwig KP, Panhuyzen-Goedkoop N, Pisani A, Solberg E, van-Buuren F, Vanhees L. Recommendations for competitive sports participation in athletes with cardiovascular disease. A consensus document from the Study Group of Sports Cardiology of the Working Group of Cardiac Rehabilitation and Exercise Physiology, and the Working Group of Myocardial and Pericardial Diseases of the European Society of Cardiology. Eur Heart J 2005, 26:1422−1445
2. Maron BJ, Zipes DP. Thirty-sixth Bethesda Conference: Eligibility Recommendations for Competitive Athletes with Cardiovascular Abnormalities. J Am Coll Cardiol 2005, 45:2−64
3. Maron BJ. Hypertrophic cardiomyopathy: a systematic review. JAMA 2002, 287:1308−1320
4. Maron BJ. Sudden death in young athletes. N Engl J Med 2003, 349:1064−1075
5. Maron BJ, Pelliccia A. The heart of trained athletes: cardiac remodelling and the risks of sports, including sudden death. Circulation 2006, 114:1633−1644

Chapter 29
Competitive Cyclist Suffering from Myocardial Infarction, Willing to Resume Competitive Sport

Mats Börjesson

Family and Personal History

This is a 44-year-old male, with no known congenital or other cardiovascular diseases in the family. No known cases of premature (<50 years) sudden cardiac death among close relatives. No known risk factors for cardiovascular disease and he denied any drugs abuse.

Athletic History

The patient had participated in leisure-time sport activities for many years, including tennis and squash. He also participated in bicycle races for many years, but not at elite level. However, during the previous 6 years the patient had spent progressively more time in bicycle training and during the 3 years he had started to be engaged at competitive level in national and international bicycle races.

Medical History

In the summer of 2006, he participated in a race in Italy lasting for several, consecutive days. He had been racing for 4 days without symptoms. On the 5th day, the weather was extremely hot and the course of the race was particularly tough with a climb up to 2400 m. During the greater part of the race the heart rate (as monitored by a Polar device) was quite high, and above 160 bpm for most of the time (Fig. 29.1). The patient felt tired, but not unusually for such an extreme race day. After 6 hours the patient reached the finishing line.

Just after the race he experienced a centrally located chest pain, and was transferred to the local hospital. He developed a myocardial infarction and subsequently

M. Börjesson (✉)
Department of Medicine, Sahlgrenska University Hospital/Östra, Göteborg, Sweden
e-mail: mats.brjesson@telia.com

A. Pelliccia (ed.), *Sports Cardiology Casebook*,
DOI 10.1007/978-1-84882-042-5_29, © Springer-Verlag London Limited 2009

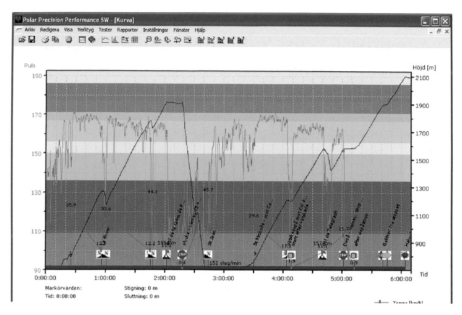

Fig. 29.1 Polar pulse watch data during the race that preceded the myocardial infarct (MI). The patient's pulse as well as the height topography of the course is outlined for the duration of the race. Pulse data is missing for the last 1 hour of the race. Mean pulse during race: 154 bpm (max 172 bpm), temperature 17–28 °C

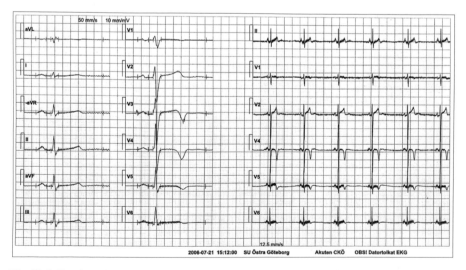

Fig. 29.2 Resting ECG 1 month post-MI. Negative T-waves are present in precordial leads V3–V5

went through a coronary angiography, which raised the need for percutaneous angio-plasty and stent placement in the left anterior descending (LAD) coronary artery.

The patient was put on standard medical treatment, including a low dose of beta-blockers (metoprolol, 50 mg daily), aspirin, clopidogrel and statins. Thorough laboratory investigation could not reveal hypercholesterolemia. The patient remained free of symptoms in the following months back home in Sweden, except for minor complaints such as atypical chest pain. The ECG showed negative T-waves, secondary to the previous infarction, in precordial leads V3–V5 (Fig. 29.2). He was referred by his doctor for new coronary angiographies twice in the subsequent months, both being perfectly normal.

The patient started exercise training again, and after some months he was able to train every day at nearly the same level as before the myocardial infarction. He did not refer any symptoms, although he could describe that his maximal pulse was 15–20 bpm lower after having started beta-blocker treatment.

Reason for Cardiovascular Evaluation

This athlete was referred for secondary opinion regarding eligibility for resumption of competitive bicycling activity. The patient was feeling well and was extremely motivated to start cycling again at a competitive level.

Physical Examination

The physical examination showed normal findings on heart and lung auscultation. The resting pulse was 52 bpm. The blood pressure was 115/60 mmHg.

12-Lead ECG

The ECG pattern was perfectly normal, showing a sinus rhythm of 52 bpm (Fig. 29.3).

Evaluation and Risk Stratification

According to the recommendations of the ESC [1] in patients with known coronary artery disease, the athlete underwent exercise ECG, echocardiography, and ECG Holter monitoring. Coronary angiography had been already performed.

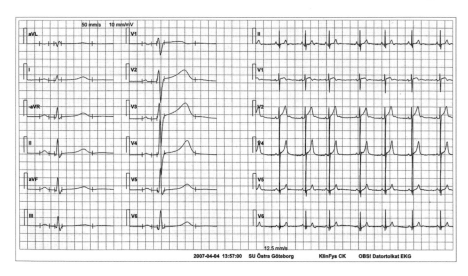

Fig. 29.3 Resting 12-lead ECG 9 months post-MI. The ECG pattern is normalized

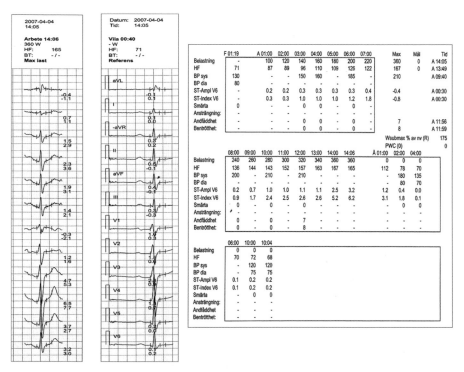

Fig. 29.4 Exercise testing performed 9 months post-MI. A maximal pulse of 167 bpm is reached, without signs of myocardial ischemia during a symptom-free test. Maximal blood pressure is 210 mmHg

Diagnostic Testing

At referral to our hospital the patient underwent a maximal symptom-limited exercise test on bicycle. The preferred method of exercise testing in Sweden is bicycle testing, which in this case was especially appropriate, since cycling was the sport of the patient. The patient was able to pedal until achieving a work load of 360 W, without symptoms and with maximal heart rate of 167 bpm (with beta-blockade) and systolic blood pressure of 210 mmHg. The electrocardiographic pattern during exercise was normal, showing no signs of myocardial ischemia (Fig. 29.4).

On echocardiography, the left ventricle was of normal dimensions, with normal systolic function (EF = 60%), in the absence of wall motion abnormalities. Diastolic function was normal on Doppler echocardiography. The patient had already been subjected to two coronary angiographies 3 and 5 months post-infarction, both showing normal results.

Recommendations

In accord to recommendations of the ESC [1] the patient was advised not to engage in competitive sports activity such as race cycling. However, he was encouraged to engage regularly in leisure-time sport, including bicycling at a safe level.

Discussion

The recommendations for eligibility in competitive sports by the European Society of Cardiology [2] state that athletes with a known coronary artery disease should refrain from competitive sport activities classified as medium-high static and medium-high dynamic. Cycle racing is actually high-intensity, high-dynamic sport activity, class III-C according to classifications in the US and Europe [2].

On assessing the different issues surrounding this decision, we considered that the patient had suffered a myocardial infarction after an exhaustive race and after several days of maximal effort in unusual climatic conditions. The first coronary angiography performed after the event showed a significant stenosis in the LAD coronary artery that was stented with success, and subsequent coronary angiographies were "normal". We do not know the specific mechanisms behind his infarction and also we do not know to what extent the sport activity may had contributed to trigger the events leading to myocardial infarction. However, we cannot exclude that the extreme conditions related to the race and weather (exhaustion, hot climate, dehydration) may have significantly contributed to this event.

Although the common laboratory results failed to show any abnormalities, we cannot exclude any existing predisposing factors (such as abnormality in the coagulability) in this patient that might had contributed to development of myocardial infarction in association with the strenuous exercise and adverse weather conditions.

Continued sport activity at the competitive level will necessarily require the capability to reach, and maintain for prolonged time periods, the maximum cardiovascular performance which results in very high heart rate and large myocardial oxygen consumption. For this reason, it seems reasonable to avoid the unnecessary risk associated with high intensive training and competitions and restrict the sport activity of this post-MI patient to leisure time activity, which may offer the several benefits of regular exercise, thereby reducing the hazards related to competitive sport.

References

1. Borjesson M, Assanelli D, Carre F, Dugmore D, Panhuysen–Goedkoop N, Seiler C, Senden J, Solberg EE. Position paper, ESC Study Group of Sports Cardiology: recommendation for participation in leisure–time physical activity and competitive sports for patients with ischaemic heart sisease. Eur J Cardiovasc Prev Rehab 2006, 13:137–149
2. Pelliccia A, Fagard R, Bjørnstad HH, Anastassakis A, Arbustini E, Assanelli D, Biffi A, Borjesson M, Carrè F, Corrado D, Delise P, Dorwarth U, Hirth A, Heidbuchel H, Hoffmann E, Mellwig KP, Panhuyzen-Goedkoop N, Pisani A, Solberg E, van-Buuren F, Vanhees L. Recommendations for competitive sports participation in athletes with cardiovascular disease. A consensus document from the Study Group of Sports Cardiology of the Working Group of Cardiac Rehabilitation and Exercise Physiology, and the Working Group of Myocardial and Pericardial Diseases of the European Society of Cardiology. Eur Heart J 2005, 26:1422–1445

Chapter 30
A 32 Year-Old Male Soccer Player with Chest Trauma

Deodato Assanelli, Evasio Pasini, Federica Ettori, Silvana Archetti, and Sabrina Arondi

Medical History

This is a 32-year-old male patient, who was non-obese, asymptomatic for angina, and a former smoker. Blood testing recently performed showed borderline total cholesterol level (210 mg/dL). The patient was a non-competitive soccer player with a training schedule of 6 h a week. The family history was positive for ischemic heart disease and deep venous thrombosis.

Physical Examination

The physical examination was negative. The blood pressure was 130±85 mmHg.

12-Lead ECG

The 12-lead ECG was normal.

Clinical Course

In the period following cardiac evaluation, the patient had a thoracic trauma (a kick in the sternum), with fast insurgence of chest pain, during a soccer match. The player was admitted to the emergency room and treated for thoracic trauma.

D. Assanelli (✉)
Chair of Sport Medicine, Department of Surgical and Medical Sciences, University of Brescia, Montichiari Hospital Via Ciotti 154, PC 25018 Montichiari, Brescia, Italy
e-mail: assanell@med.unibs.it

A. Pelliccia (ed.), *Sports Cardiology Casebook*,
DOI 10.1007/978-1-84882-042-5_30, © Springer-Verlag London Limited 2009

Cardiac Evaluation in the CCU

Seven day later, the patient was admitted again to the coronary care unit (CCU) because of acute pain in the right mammary region, radiating to the right shoulder, lasting for 2 h. A new ECG was recorded which showed signs of myocardial ischemia, as illustrated in Fig. 30.1. In addition, elevated blood level of myocardial enzymes was found (CPK = 3469 U/L, CPK-MB = 460 ng/mL). An echocardiogram was promptly performed showing akinesia of LV antero-lateral wall. Then coronary angiography (Fig. 30.2) was performed, which showed thrombotic

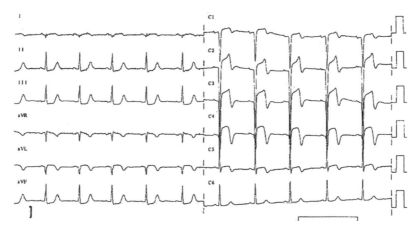

Fig. 30.1 ECG performed after thoracic trauma. The signs of myocardial ischemia are evident, as shown by the ST segment elevation in the precordial leads V1∓V5, and standard leads I and aVL, with inverted T wave most prominent in leads V3∓V5 and aVL. Correspondingly, ST segment depression is present in standard leads II, III and aVF

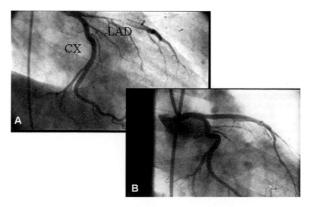

Fig. 30.2 Coronary angiography of the same athlete, showing occlusion of the proximal and intermediate left anterior descending (LAD) coronary artery (**a**). Consequently, PTCA was performed and stent implanted, with resumed blood flow into LAD coronary artery (**b**)

occlusion of the proximal and intermediate left anterior descending coronary artery. Consequently, PTCA was performed and a stent was implanted. The procedure was well tolerated but LV systolic function remained depressed (ejection fraction: 30%). Two days later, the patient had also a transitory ischemic attack (TIA), but recovered promptly.

Additional Testing

Considering the low risk profile for ischemic heart disease, the positive family history for vascular disease and the severity of clinical course in this patient, we analyzed specific vascular risk factors. The patient was found to be homozygous for the G1691A mutation of clotting factor V gene and for C667T (principal MTFR mutation). He also had an apo4 allele (3/4) and high homocysteine (32 μmol/L).

Recommendations

The international recommendations for eligibility in competitive sports published by the European Society of Cardiology [1, 2] state that athletes with a known coronary artery disease should refrain from competitive sport activities classified as medium-high static and medium-high dynamic. The patient was advised therefore not to be engaged in competitive soccer. However, he was encouraged to be regularly engaged in leisure-time sport, such as jogging, swimming or bicycling at a safe level.

Discussion

The clinical case here brings a specific message: that in all subjects with acute chest pain, the presence of myocardial ischemia should be considered and appropriately excluded. In addition, when coronary artery disease is found in young persons (<35 years), careful search for additional risk factors is advisable, specifically if the family history is positive. The player in this case had a low risk profile for ischemic heart disease, was young, a non-smoker, with a normal blood pressure and only borderline cholesterol level. However, the severity of the clinical course and the positive family history raised suspicion for other (vascular) risk factors, which were eventually confirmed by findings of two (genetically inherited) pro-thrombotic conditions (high homocysteine and homozygous V Leiden factor).

References

1. Pelliccia A, Fagard R, Bjørnstad HH, Anastassakis A, Arbustini E, Assanelli D, Biffi A, Borjesson M, Carrè F, Corrado D, Delise P, Dorwarth U, Hirth A, Heidbuchel H, Hoffmann E, Mellwig KP, Panhuyzen-Goedkoop N, Pisani A, Solberg E, van-Buuren F, Vanhees L.

Recommendations for competitive sports participation in athletes with cardiovascular disease. A consensus document from the Study Group of Sports Cardiology of the Working Group of Cardiac Rehabilitation and Exercise Physiology, and the Working Group of Myocardial and Pericardial Diseases of the European Society of Cardiology. Eur Heart J 2005, 26:1422–1445

2. Börjesson M, Assanelli D, Carre' F, Dugmore D, Panhuyzen–Goedkoop NM, Seiler C, Senden J, Solberg EE. ESC Study Group of Sports Cardiology:recommendations for participation in leisure–time physical activity and competitive sports for patients with ischaemic heart disease. Eur J Cardiovasc Prev Rehab 2006, 13:137–149

Chapter 31
Asymptomatic Cyclist with Stenosis of Left Main Coronary Artery

Deodato Assanelli, Enrico Ballardini, Evasio Pasini, Giancarlo Magri, and Sabrina Arondi

Medical History

This is a 53-year-old, asymptomatic, male patient. He was obese, and smoked 15 cigarettes a day. In recent blood analysis, a modest hypercholesterolemia (225 mg/dL, HDL-C 52, LDL-C 149) was documented. The family history was positive for systemic hypertension and ischemic heart disease. Patient participated in many leisure-time sport activities. In the last years, however, he spent progressively more time in non-competitive bicycle racing by training about 8 h a week.

Physical Examination

Cardiac physical examination was negative; blood pressure was 140–100 mmHg

12-Lead ECG

The 12-lead ECG was normal (Fig. 31.1).

Exercise Testing

Considering the high risk profile and high level of sport activity, exercise testing was performed to assess the occurrence of any change suggestive for ischemic heart disease. The test was submaximal and the patient stopped because of muscular fatigue at 85% of estimated maximal heart rate. The patient remained completely asymptomatic and the test was considered negative for inducible myocardial ischemia (Fig. 31.2).

D. Assanelli (✉)
Chair of Sport Medicine, Department of Surgical and Medical Sciences, University of Brescia, Montichiari Hospital Via Ciotti 154, PC 25018 Montichiari, Brescia, Italy
e-mail: assanell@med.unibs.it

A. Pelliccia (ed.), *Sports Cardiology Casebook*,
DOI 10.1007/978-1-84882-042-5_31, © Springer-Verlag London Limited 2009

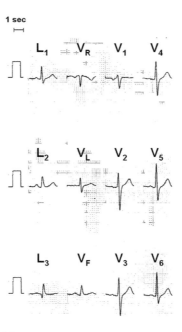

Fig. 31.1 Resting 12-lead ECG

Additional Testing

However, the presence of a positive family history and multiple risk factors suggested, at the occasion of a subsequent medical check up, a repeat of the exercise testing until exhaustion.

At the peak of the new exercise test, we observed marked ST-segment depressions up to 3 mm in the precordial leads V4, V5 and V6, which slowly disappeared during the recovery (Fig. 31.3).

Despite marked ECG changes, the subject had remained asymptomatic for the entire duration of the test. Subsequently, myocardial perfusion scintigraphy was performed (Fig. 31.4), which confirmed the occurrence of reversible reduced perfusion in the inferior and lateral LV wall. The patient underwent coronary angiography, which confirmed the presence of a significant stenosis of the left main coronary artery (Fig. 31.5).

Diagnosis and Recommendations

The patient had silent ischemia due to coronary artery disease, affecting primarily the left main coronary artery. The case was discussed with surgeons and a surgical revascularisation was advised. Patient received three coronary by-passes. During the post-operative period he had no complications and successfully performed a rehabilitation program. After a few months he resumed non-competitive sport, without

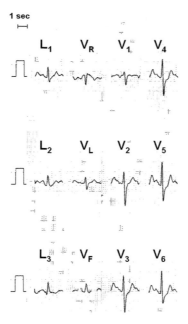

Fig. 31.2 ECG recorded during sub-maximal exercise testing: mild ST segment changes were observed, judged to be not suggestive for myocardial ischemia

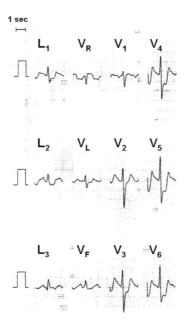

Fig. 31.3 ECG recorded during maximal exercise test showed significant ST segment depression in precordial leads V4, V5, V6, suggestive for myocardial ischemia

Fig. 31.4 Myocardial perfusion scintigraphy after maximal exercise test showed reversible reduced perfusion in the inferior and lateral LV wall

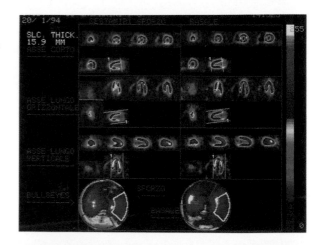

Fig. 31.5 Coronary angiography. A stenosis of the left main coronary artery was found

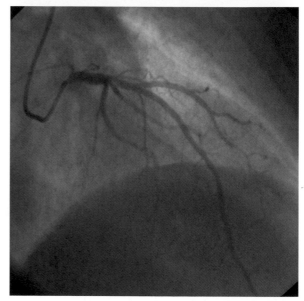

symptoms or any limitations. At present, he is regularly cycling without symptoms or limitations, and periodical (annual) clinical follow-ups, including exercise ECG, remained normal.

Discussion

This clinical case illustrated above conveys a specific message: in a subject with high risk for ischemic heart disease who performs regular and intense physical activity, in spite of absence of symptoms, a maximal exercise test should be performed [1, 2].

In fact, in this patient who had significant coronary artery disease, a sub-maximal exercise was negative and potentially misjudging. The maximal exercise testing may allow timely identification of silent coronary disease in athletic patients, thus starting therapeutic procedures and avoiding the occurrence adverse clinical events.

References

1. Pelliccia A, Fagard R, Bjørnstad HH, Anastassakis A, Arbustini E, Assanelli D, Biffi A, Borjesson M, Carrè F, Corrado D, Delise P, Dorwarth U, Hirth A, Heidbuchel H, Hoffmann E, Mellwig KP, Panhuyzen-Goedkoop N, Pisani A, Solberg E, van-Buuren F, Vanhees L. Recommendations for competitive sports participation in athletes with cardiovascular disease. A consensus document from the Study Group of Sports Cardiology of the Working Group of Cardiac Rehabilitation and Exercise Physiology, and the Working Group of Myocardial and Pericardial Diseases of the European Society of Cardiology. Eur Heart J 2005, 26:1422–1445
2. Börjesson M, Assanelli D, Carrè F, Dugmore D, Panhuyzen-Goedkoop NM, Seiler C, Sender J, Solberg EE. ESC Study Group of Sports Cardiology; recommendations for participation in leisure- time physical activity and competitive sports for patients with is chaemic heart disease. Eur J Cardiovasc Prev Rehab 2006, 13:137–149

Appendices

Appendix A Classification of Sports[§]

	A. Low dynamic	B. Moderate dynamic	C. High dynamic
I. Low Static	Archery Bowling Cricket Golf Rifle	Table tennis Tennis (doubles) Volleyball Baseball*	Badminton Walking Running (marathon) Cross-country skiing (classic)
II. Moderate Static	Auto racing*~ Diving~ Equestrian*~ Motorcycling*~ Gymnastics* Karate/Judo* Sailing	Fencing Field events (jumping) Figure skating* Lacrosse* Running (sprint)	Basketball* Biathlon Ice hockey* Field hockey* Football* Soccer* Cross-country skiing (skating) Running (middle/ long distance) Swimming Squash* Tennis (single) Team handball*
III. High Static	Bobsledding *~ Field events (throwing) Luge*~ Rock Climbing*~ Waterskiing*~ Weight lifting* Windsurfing*~	Body building* Downhill skiing*~ Wrestling*	Boxing* Canoeing, Kayaking Cycling*~ Decathlon Rowing Speed skating

Symbols: *Danger of bodily collision.
~Increased risk if syncope occurs.
§ Adapted and modified after Mitchell et al. (Classification of Sports. JACC 1994, 24:864–866).

Appendix B Recommendations for Competitive Sport Participation in Athletes with Congenital Heart Diseases

Lesion	Evaluation	Criteria for eligibility	Recommendation	Follow-up
Atrial septal defect (closed or small, unoperated) and patent foramen oOvale	History, NYHA functional class, PE, ECG, echo, chest X-ray, ET	<6 mm defect, or 6 months postclosure, with normal pulmonary artery pressure, no significant arrhythmia or ventricular dysfunction	All sports In patients with PFO percutaneous closure may be considered before regular scubadiving	Yearly
Ventricular septal defect (closed or small unoperated)	History, NYHA functional class, PE, ECG, echo, chest X-ray, ET	Restrictive defect (left-to-right gradient >64 mmHg) or 6 months postclosure, no pulmonary hypertension	All sports	Yearly
Atrioventricular septal defect	History, NYHA functional class, PE, ECG, echo, chest X-ray, ET	No or only mild AV valve insufficiency, no significant subaortic stenosis or arrhythmia, normal maximal gas exchange measurements	All sports	Yearly. Complete reassessment every 2nd year
Partial or complete Anomalous Pulmonary Venous Connection	History, NYHA functional class, PE, ECG, echo, chest X-ray, ET, MRI	No significant pulmonary or systemic venous obstruction, no pulmonary hypertension or exercise-induced atrial arrhythmia	All sports	Yearly
Persistent ductus Arteriosus (operated)	History, NYHA functional class, PE, ECG, echo, chest X-ray, ET	Six months postclosure and no residual pulmonary hypertension	All sports	Not needed
Pulmonary stenosis (mild native or treated)	History, NYHA functional class, PE, ECG, echo, chest X-ray, ET	Native or 6 months postinterventional/ postsurgical; peak transvalvular gradient <30 mmHg, normal RV, normal ECG or only mild RV hypertrophy, no significant arrhythmias	All sports	Yearly

Appendix B (continued)

Lesion	Evaluation	Criteria for eligibility	Recommendation	Follow-up
Pulmonary stenosis (moderate native or treated)	History, NYHA functional class, PE, ECG, echo, chest X-ray, ET	Native or 6 months postinterventional/postsurgical; peak transvalvular gradient between 30 and 50 mmHg, normal RV, normal ECG or only mild RV hypertrophy	Low and moderate dynamic and low static sport (I A,B)	Every 6 months
Coarctation of the aorta (native or repaired)	History, NYHA functional class, PE, ECG, echo, chest X-ray, ET, MRI	No systemic hypertension; peak pressure gradient between the upper and lower limbs of <21 mmHg, a peak systolic BP during exercise of <231 mmHg, no ischemia on exercise ECG, no left ventricular overload	Low and moderate dynamic and static sport (I, II A, B) If interposed graft avoid sport with a risk of bodily collision	Yearly. Complete reassessment every 2nd year
Aortic stenosis (mild)	History, NYHA functional class, PE, ECG, echo, chest X-ray, ET	Mean transvalvular gradient <21 mmHg, no history of arrhythmia, no syncope, dizziness or angina pectoris	All sports, with exception of high static, high dynamic sports	Yearly
Aortic stenosis (moderate)	History, NYHA functional class, PE, ECG, echo, chest X-ray, ET, 24-h Holter	Mean transvalvular gradient between 21 and 49 mmHg, no history of arrhythmia, no syncope, dizziness or angina pectoris	Low dynamic and static sport (I A)	Every 6 months

Appendix B (continued)

Lesion	Evaluation	Criteria for eligibility	Recommendation	Follow-up
Tetralogy of Fallot	History, NYHA functional class, PE, ECG, echo, chest X-ray, ET, 24-h Holter, MRI	Non or only mild RVOT obstruction, no more than mild pulmonary regurgitation, a normal or near normal biventricular function and no evidence of arrhythmia Moderate residual lesion with RV pressure <50% of systemic pressure, or residual VSD or moderate pulmonary regurgitation, but normal biventricular function	Low and moderate static and dynamic sport. (I, II A, B) Low static and dynamic sport. (I A) Patients with conduit should avoid sport with risk of bodily collision	Yearly. Complete reassessment every 2nd year
Transposition of the great arteries (arterial switch)	History, NYHA functional class, PE, ECG, echo, chest X-ray, ET	No or only mild neo-aortic insufficiency, no significant pulmonary stenosis, no signs of ischemia or arrhythmia on exercise ECG	All sports, with exception of high static, high dynamic sports	Yearly

Abbreviations: ECG = 12-lead electrocardiogram; ET = exercise testing; Echo = echocardiography; PE = physical examination; MRI = cardiac magnetic resonance imaging; 24-h Holter = 24 h Holter ECG monitoring
Follow-up includes medical record, NYHA functional class, PE, ECG, echo. Supplementary investigation will be performed dependent on lesion and symptoms

Appendix C Recommendations for Competitive Sport Participation in Athletes with Valvular Disease

Lesion	Evaluation	Criteria for eligibility	Recommendations	Follow-up
Mitral valve stenosis	History, PE, ECG, ET, echo	Mild stenosis, stable sinus rhythm	All sports, with exception of high dynamic and high static (III C)	Yearly
		Mild stenosis in atrial fibrillation, and anticoagulation	Low-moderate dynamic, low-moderate static (I–II, A, B). No contact sport	Yearly
		Moderate and severe stenosis (atrial fibrillation or sinus rhythm)	Low dynamic and low static (IA) No contact sport	Yearly
Mitral valve regurgitation	History, PE, ECG, ET, echo	Mild to moderate regurgitation, stable sinus rhythm, normal LV size/function, normal exercise testing	All sports	Yearly
		Mild to moderate regurgitation, normal LV size and function, normal exercise testing. If atrial fibrillation, in anticoagulation	All sports, with exception of contact sport	Yearly
		Mild to moderate regurgitation, mild LV dilatation (end-systolic volume <55 mL/m^2), normal LV function, in sinus rhythm	Low-moderate dynamic, low-moderate static (I–II, A,B)	Yearly
		Mild to moderate regurgitation, LV enlargement (end-systolic volume >55 mL/m^2) or LV dysfunction (ejection fraction <50%)	No competitive sports	
		Severe regurgitation	No competitive sports	

Appendix C (continued)

Lesion	Evaluation	Criteria for eligibility	Recommendations	Follow-up
Aortic valve stenosis	History, PE, ECG, ET, echo	Mild stenosis, normal LV size and function at rest and under stress, no symptoms, no significant arrhythmia	Low-moderate dynamic, low-moderate static (I–II, A,B)	Yearly
		Moderate stenosis, normal LV function at rest and under stress, frequent/complex arrhythmias	Low dynamic and low static (IA)	Yearly
		Moderate stenosis, LV dysfunction at rest or under stress, symptoms	No competitive sports	
		Severe stenosis	No competitive sports	
Aortic valve regurgitation	History, PE, ECG, ET, echo	Mild to moderate regurgitation, normal LV size and function, normal exercise testing, no significant arrhythmia	All sports	Yearly
		Mild to moderate regurgitation, proof of progressive LV dilatation	Low dynamic and low static (IA)	Yearly
		Mild to moderate regurgitation, significant ventricular arrhythmia at rest or under stress, dilatation of the ascending aorta	No competitive sports	
		Severe regurgitation	No competitive sports	
Tricuspid valve stenosis	History, PE, ECG, ET, echo	No symptoms	Low-moderate dynamic, low-moderate static (I–II, A,B)	Every 2nd year

Appendix C (continued)

Lesion	Evaluation	Criteria for eligibility	Recommendations	Follow-up
Tricuspid valve regurgitation	History, PE, ECG, ET, echo	Mild to moderate regurgitation	Low-moderate dynamic, low-moderate static (I-II, A – B)	Yearly
		Any degree, with right atrial pressure more than 20 mmHg	No competitive sports	
Poly-valvular diseases	History, PE, ECG, ET, echo		see most relevant defect	
Bioprosthetic aortic or mitral valve	History, PE, ECG, ET, echo	Normal valve function and normal LV function, in stable sinus rhythm	Low-moderate dynamic, low-moderate static (I–II, A,B)	Yearly
		Normal valve function and normal LV function, in atrial fibrillation	Low-moderate dynamic, low-moderate static (I–II, A,B) No contact types of sport	Yearly
Prosthetic (artificial) aortic or mitral valve	History, PE, ECG, ET, echo	Normal valve function and normal LV function, and anticoagulation	Low-moderate dynamic, low-moderate static (I–II, A,B) No contact types of sport	Yearly
Post valvuloplasty	History, PE, ECG, ET, echo	See the residual severity of the mitral valve stenosis or mitral valve regurgitation	Low-moderate dynamic, low-moderate static (I–II, A,B) No contact types of sport	Yearly
Mitral valve prolapse	History, PE, ECG, ET, echo	If unexplained syncope, or family history of sudden death, or complex supraventricular or ventricular arrhythmias, or long QT interval or severe mitral regurgitation	No competitive sports	
		Absence of the above cited cases	All sports	Yearly

Abbreviations: ECG: 12-lead electrocardiography; Echo = Echocardiography; ET:exercise stress testing; PE = physical examination; Sport type: see Appendix A.

Appendix D Recommendation for Competitive Sport Participation in Athletes with Cardiomyopathies, Myocarditis and Pericarditis

Lesion	Evaluation	Criteria for eligibility	Recommendations	Follow-up
Athletes with definite diagnosis of HCM	History, PE, ECG echo		No competitive sports	
Athletes with definite diagnosis of HCM but low risk profile	History, PE, ECG, echo, ET, 24-h Holter	No SD in the relatives, no symptoms; mild LVH, normal BP response to exercise; no ventricular arrhythmias	Low dynamic, low static sports (I A)	Yearly
Athletes with only gene abnormalities of HCM, without phenotype changes	History, PE, ECG, echo	No symptoms, no LVH, no ventricular arrhythmias	Only recreational, non-competitive sport activities	Yearly
Athletes with definite diagnosis of DCM	History, PE, ECG, echo		No competitive sports	
Athletes with definite diagnosis of DCM but low risk profile	History, PE, ECG, echo, ET, 24-h Holter	No SD in the relatives, no symptoms; mildly depressed EF ($\geq$40%), normal BP response to exercise; no complex ventricular arrhythmias	Low-moderate dynamic and low static sports (IA, IB)	Yearly
Athletes with definite diagnosis of ARVC	History, PE, ECG echo		No competitive sports	
Athletes with active myocarditis, or pericarditis	History, PE, ECG, echo		No competitive sports	
Athletes after resolution of myocarditis	History, PE, ECG, echo, ET	No symptoms, normal LV function, no arrhythmias	All competitive sports	1st control within 6 months*
Athletes after resolution of pericarditis	History, PE, ECG, echo, ET	No symptoms, normal LV function, No arrhythmias	All competitive sports	1st control within 6 months*

Abbreviations: ARVC = arrhythmogenic right ventricular cardiomyopathy; BP = blood pressure; DCM = dilated cardiomyopathy; HCM = hypertrophic cardiomyopathy; Echo = Echocardiography; EF = ejection fraction; ET = Exercise testing; 24-h Holter: 24-h Holter ECG monitoring; LV = left ventricular; LVH = left ventricular hypertrophy; PE physical examination; SD = sudden death; Sport type, see Appendix A.
* Subsequent controls according to the individual case.

Appendix E   Recommendation for Competitive Sport Participation in Athletes with Marfan's Syndrome

Phenotype	Genotype	Criteria for eligibility	Recommendations	Follow-up
Adult with full phenotype; adolescent with incomplete phenotype; children/adolescent without phenotype	Positive		No competitive sports	
Athletes (adults) with full phenotype	Not available		No competitive sports	
Athletes (adolescents) with incomplete phenotype	Not available	Positive family history	No competitive sports	
Athletes (adolescents) with incomplete phenotype	Not available	Negative family history	Continued sport participation with follow-up	Yearly
Athletes (children/adolescent) without phenotype	Not available	Positive family history	Continued sport participation with follow-up	Yearly

Appendix F Stratification of Risk to Quantify Prognosis in Patients with Systemic Hypertension

	Clinic blood pressure (mmHg)		
Other risk factors and disease history	Grade 1 SBP 140–159 or DBP 90–99	Grade 2 SBP 160–179 or DBP 100–109	Grade 3 SBP = 180 or DBP = 110
No other risk factors[a]	Low added risk	Moderate added risk	High added risk
1–2 risk factors[a]	Moderate added risk	Moderate added risk	Very high added risk
3 or more risk factors[a] or TOD[b] or diabetes	High added risk	High added risk	Very high added risk
Associated clinical conditions[c]	Very high added risk	Very high added risk	Very high added risk

Abbreviations: TOD = target organ damage; SBP = systolic blood pressure; DBP = diastolic blood pressure Low, moderate, high and very high added risk indicate an approximate 10-year risk of fatal and nonfatal cardiovascular disease of $<15\%$, $15–20\%$; $20–30\%$ and $>30\%$, or of fatal cardiovascular disease of $<4\%$, $4–5\%$, $5–8\%$ and $>8\%$

Symbols: [a] Risk factors used for stratification: blood pressure level (grades 1–3); gender and age (men >55 years; women >65 years); smoking; dyslipidaemia (total cholesterol >250 mg/dL or LDL-cholesterol >155 mg/dL or HDL-cholesterol <40 mg/dL in men and <48 mg/dL in women); abdominal obesity (men $=102$ cm; women $=88$ cm); 1st degree family history of premature cardiovascular disease (men <55 years; women <65 years)

[b] Target organ damage: hypertension-induced left ventricular hypertrophy; ultrasound evidence of arterial wall thickening or atherosclerotic plaque; slight increase in serum creatinine (men 1.3–1.5 mg/dL; women 1.2–1.4 mg/dL); presence of micro-albuminuria

[c] Associated clinical conditions: cerebrovascular disease; ischaemic heart disease; heart failure; peripheral vascular disease; renal impairment; proteinuria; advanced retinopathy (haemorrhages; exsudates; papiloedema)

Appendix G   Recommendation for Competitive Sport Participation in Athletes with Systemic Hypertension (and Other Risk Factors) According to the Cardiovascular Risk Profile

Lesion	Evaluation	Criteria for eligibility	Recommendations	Follow-up
Low added risk	History, PE, ECG, ET; echo	Well controlled BP	All sports	Yearly
Moderate added risk	History, PE, ECG, ET; echo	Well controlled BP and risk factors	All sports, with exclusion of high static, high dynamic sports (III C)	Yearly
High added risk	History, PE, ECG, ET; echo	Well controlled BP and risk factors	All sports, with exclusion of high static sports (III A–C)	Yearly
Very high added risk	History, PE, ECG, ET; echo	Well controlled BP and risk factors; no associated clinical conditions	Only low-moderate dynamic, low static sports (I A,B)	6 months

Abbreviations: BP = blood pressure; LVH = left ventricular hypertrophy; PE : physical examination, including repeated blood pressure measurements according to guidelines [54–57]
Symbols: [a, b, c] as in Appendix F

Appendix H Recommendation for Competitive Sport Participation in Athletes with Ischemic Heart Disease

Lesion	Evaluation	Criteria for eligibility	Recommendations	Follow-up
Athletes with definite diagnosis of IHD and high probability of cardiac events	History, ECG, ET, echo, coronary-angiography		No competitive sports allowed	
Athletes with definite diagnosis of IHD and low probability of cardiac events	History, ECG, ET, echo, coronary-angiography	No exercise induced ischemia, no symptoms or major arrhythmias, not significant (<50%) coronary lesions, EF >50%	Only low-moderate dynamic and low static sports (IA, IB)	Yearly
Athletes without evidence of IHD but with high risk profile (>5% global SCORE)	History, ECG, ET	If positive provocative ECGs, further testing are needed (stress echo, scintigraphy and/or coronary angiography) to confirm IHD. If positive, consider as athletes with diagnosis of IHD	Only low-moderate dynamic and low static sports (IA, IB)	Yearly
		If negative provocative ECGs	Individual based decision; avoid high static sports (IIIA–C)	Yearly
Athletes without evidence of IHD and low risk profile	History, ECG, ET optional	Negative ECG	All competitive sports	Every 1–3 years

Abbreviations: ECG = 12-lead electrocardiogram; ET = Exercise testing or other provocative testing; IHD = ischemic heart disease; Sport type I–III, A–C, see Appendix A

Appendix I Recommendation for Competitive Sport Participation in Athletes with Arrhythmias and Arrhythmogenic Conditions

Lesion	Evaluation	Criteria for eligibility	Recommendations	Follow-up
Marked sinus bradycardia (<40 bpm) and/or sinus pauses ≥ 3 s with symptoms	History, ECG, ET, 24-h Holter, echo	(a) If symptoms# are present (b) After >3 months from resolution of symptoms#; off therapy	(a) Temporary interruption of sport (b) All sports	Yearly
(a) A–V block 1st and 2nd degree, type 1 (b) A–V block 2nd degree, type 2 or advanced	History, ECG, ET, 24-h Holter, echo	(a) If no symptoms#, no cardiac disease, with resolution during exercise (b) In the absence of symptoms, cardiac disease, ventricular arrhythmias during exercise, and if resting heart rate is >40 bpm	(a) All sports (b) Low-moderate dynamic, low-moderate static sports (I, II A,B)	Yearly
Supraventricular premature beats	History, ECG, thyroid function	No symptoms#, no cardiac disease	All sports	Not required
Paroxysmal supraventricular tachycardia (AVNRT or AVRT over a concealed accessory pathway)	History, ECG, echo. EP study	Ablation is recommended: (a) After catheter ablation: if no recurrences for >3 months, and no cardiac disease (b) If ablation is not performed and AVNRT is sporadic, without cardiac disease, without hemodynamic consequences and without relation with exercise	(a) All sports (b) All sports, except those with increased risk	Yearly
Ventricular pre-excitation (WPW syndrome) and: (a) Paroxysmal AV reentry tachycardia (b) Atrial fibrillation or flutter (c) Asymptomatic pre-excitation pattern	(a, b,c) History, ECG, echo, EP study	(a,b) Ablation is mandatory after catheter ablation: if no recurrences, no cardiac disease (c) Ablation is recommended but not mandatory.	(a, b) All sports (c) Asymptomatic athletes at low risk and not ablated: all sports, except those with increased risk*	Yearly

Appendix I (continued)

Lesion	Evaluation	Criteria for eligibility	Recommendations	Follow-up
Atrial fibrillation (paroxysmal, permanent)	History, ECG, echo, ET, 24-h Holter	(a) After paroxysmal AF: if no cardiac disease, no WPW, and stable sinus rhythm >3 months (b) Permanent A F in the absence of cardiac disease, and WPW: assess heart rate and LV function response to exercise	(a) All sports (b) Assessed on individual basis	(a) Yearly (b) Every 6 months
Atrial flutter	History, ECG, echo, EP study	Ablation is mandatory after ablation: if no symptoms# for >3 months, no cardiac disease or WPW, and off therapy;	All sports	Yearly
Premature ventricular beats	History, ECG, echo (ET, 24-h Holter, in selected cases invasive tests)	In the absence of cardiac disease or arrhythmogenic condition^, family history of SD, symptoms#, relation with exercise, frequent and/or polymorphic PVBs and/or frequent couplets with short RR interval	All sports	Yearly
Nonsustained ventricular tachycardia	History, ECG, echo (ET, 24-h Holter, in selected cases invasive tests)	In the absence of cardiac disease or arrhythmogenic^ condition, symptoms#, family history of SD, relation with exercise, multiple episodes of NSVT with short RR interval	All sports	Every 6 months
Slow ventricular tachycardia, fascicular ventricular tachycardia, right ventricular outflow tachycardia	History, ECG, echo, ET, 24-h Holter, (in selected cases EP study)	In the absence of cardiac disease or arrhythmogenic^ condition, family history of SD, symptoms#	All sports, except those with increased risk*	Every 6 months
Syncope	History, ECG, echo, ET, 24-h Holter; tilting test	(a) Neurocardiogenic (b) Arrhythmic or primary cardiac	(a) All sports (except those with increased risk*) (b) See specific cause	Yearly

Appendix I (continued)

Lesion	Evaluation	Criteria for eligibility	Recommendations	Follow-up
Long QT syndrome	History, ECG, (24-h Holter, genetic testing)	Positive long QT syndrome	No competitive sports	
Brugada syndrome	History, ECG, provocative test	Positive Brugada syndrome	No competitive sports	
Implanted pacemaker	ECG, echo, ET, 24-h Holter	Normal heart rate increase during exercise, no significant arrhythmias, normal cardiac function	Low-moderate dynamic and low static sports (I, II A), except those with risk of bodily collision	Yearly
Implantable cardioverter defibrillator	ECG, echo, ET, 24-h Holter	No malignant VTs; normal cardiac function; at least 6 months after the implantion, or the last ICD intervention	Low-moderate dynamic and low static sports (I, II A), except those with risk of bodily collision	Yearly

Abbreviations: ECG = 12-lead electrocardiogram; Echo = echocardiography; ET = Exercise testing; 24-h Holter = 24-h Holter monitoring; EP = Electrophysiologic; Sport types, see Appendix A

Symbols: * increased risk if syncope occurs (see Classification of Sports);

\# symptoms include presyncope, lightheadedness, exertional fatigue;

^ arrhythmogenic conditions include cardiomyopathies, ischemic heart disease and channelopathies

NB. For athletes with structural heart disease, see the recommendations of the disease

Index

Printed in the United States of America

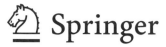 Springer